IT'S JUST NERVES

Burn This House

IT'S JUST NERVES
notes on a disability

KELLY DAVIO

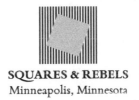

SQUARES & REBELS
Minneapolis, Minnesota

COPYRIGHT

Squares & Rebels
PO Box 3941
Minneapolis, MN 55403-0941
E-mail: squaresandrebels@gmail.com
Online: squaresandrebels.com

Printed in the United States of America.
ISBN: 978-1-941960-06-6
Library of Congress Control Number: 2017936469

A Squares & Rebels First Edition

CONTENTS

IV. The Wide World

for

Steve Cook

Those who be in trouble with a scarcity of spirits, are able at first rising in the morning to walk, move their arms this way and that, or to lift up a weight with strength; but before noon, the stores of spirits which influenced the muscles being almost spent, they are scarce able to move hand or foot. I now have a prudent and honest woman in cure, who for many years has been obnoxious to this kind of bastard palsy not only in the limbs, but likewise in her tongue; this person for some time speaks freely and readily enough, but after long, hasty, or laborious speaking, she becomes mute as a fish and cannot bring forth a word, nay, and does not recover the use of her voice till after an hour or two.

—first documented description of myasthenia gravis,
by Thomas Willis in *De anima Brutorum*, 1672

I. THE MIRROR

STRONG IS THE NEW SEXY

In the hospital complex, I sit in a room with a woman who plans to teach me how to swallow. Or, to re-teach me. I knew how to swallow just as I knew how to breathe. It's just that, somewhere along the way, my body's muscles have forgotten.

The physical therapist holds a stethoscope to my throat and listens to me sip ice water. Some time later we move to applesauce, then to a dry and crumbling cracker. She makes notes on a clipboard, studies them.

On the other side of the plate-glass window of the physical therapy room, hang gliders swoop down from the pine-covered mountainside. Their sails are the bright neon of 1990s fashion, and it's impossible to miss the daredevils with their spectacular, spandexed bodies. I wonder whether the location of the window is intended to be inspirational: a call to the possibilities of good health, a motivation to perform one's exercises well and *get back out there*. I have an impulse to drop the blinds over the window. I'd like to occlude the mountain.

I used to grade student papers in waiting rooms, but my red pen and a sheaf of student essays invited too many comments from others—where did I teach, what grade level, did I enjoy my work. On such occasions, I prefer to keep my own counsel. I have developed the habit of pulling out my smart phone and flipping mindlessly through applications, dissolving the minutes ahead of my appointments for which I always seem to arrive early.

I open an application called Pinterest. It's a perfectly innocuous, time-wasting service that shows me photos of things that my friends enjoy. I scroll through images of dogs lolling on grass, craft projects that no one I know has the time or skill to complete, aspirational home renovation schemes. My thumb whisks the world by at a clip or a crawl; I am all-powerful on this tiniest of screens.

Scrolling through this array of images, I know I run the risk of seeing it. I know that I should stop while my mind is full of photos of captioned

3

housecats and decorated cookies, but I scroll on. And there it is, a photo of a gorgeous, well-fed, hourglass-figured girl stepping from the ocean in a bandeau bikini. The caption that hovers below her, as though emerging from the sand, reads: "Being healthy and fit is so much more important than being skinny."

The physical therapist lifts her head from her notes to tell me that she cannot assign me any exercises. They're very effective for most people, she says. Science has the data to prove it. Yet it's the nature of my condition, she reminds me, that with attempts at repeated movement, my body will rush antibodies to the site where nerve meets muscle, the immune system blocking the neurotransmitters. Repeated flexing will only make my muscles weaker. We are going to focus instead, she says, on "technique."

She shows me how to tuck my chin to my chest as I swallow. This will keep me from aspirating my food, and from sucking water down my windpipe and into my lungs. On a paper handout that has been photocopied many times over, its text grown fuzzy over time, she shows me a cross-section of the human chest, points to where food particles can land in the bronchial tree, and explains that pneumonia flourishes on their half-chewed surfaces.

She demonstrates how to hold my head at an angle as I chew, as though I were casually glancing over my shoulder as I masticate another cracker. This posture is meant to block the weaker side of my throat and keep me from choking. It's hard to imagine doing this at home on a regular basis, much less making a go of this chin-tuck and shoulder-glance attitude at a nice restaurant (*what's that woman looking at?*) but I do as she asks.

The most important thing, she tells me, is that I don't quit eating. Sometimes people just give up, she says. She looks at my chart again, and asks how much weight I've lost in the past few months.

The product of a generation of girls who grew up with the specter of anorexia stalking our friends and siblings, I was told that "real women have curves" as though it were a mantra.

Our elders were trying. They wanted to flip the arbitrary concept of thin-body beauty on its ear. They wanted us to find self-acceptance, but when they tried to scare us with photos of undernourished bodies and cautionary tales of the dangers of disordered eating, we learned that being skinny was one more way in which we could fail—one more way our bodies could be repellant.

With the onset of a progressive neuromuscular disease several years ago, my body's relationship with solid food became a complicated one. I was never a curvy woman to begin with, but with each of the more feminine attributes I've lost, I've become, I am given to understand, less and less of a real woman.

I wonder at what point I will become unreal altogether.

At first it was easy enough to cover for some of the effects of my illness under the guise of sheer clumsiness. I dropped things, I stumbled, and sometimes I garbled my words, but I was never an elegant, balletic woman. Known for knocking over glasses of water or tripping over the smallest of cracks in the sidewalk, I was happy enough to chalk my bungled movements up to idiosyncrasy. For a couple of years I could pass for a real woman.

By their nature, progressive diseases worsen over time. I stopped breathing now and then. Chewing was a hit-and-miss proposition. Sipping water became, at times, more trouble than it was worth; to a weakened arm, a bottle of spring water is as hard to raise as a dumbbell.

I began to lack reality. I took to baggy tops and A-line silhouettes to hide my poking collarbone, my meatless hips. I took up as much space as I could in bulky sweaters. I compensated for my diminishing reality by covering over my negative space.

As I sit in the therapy room, waiting while my therapist gathers papers, pamphlets, and documents of all sorts from the hospital's cavernous hall, I take to my phone and scroll. I scroll almost compulsively, as if distraction with images of lovely shoes and frosted cakes and gamboling baby ducklings were the same thing as comfort.

I see another picture, one of a woman with a muscle-bound, thong-clad butt. The caption above her grayscale image tells me what I already suspect to be true: "Strong is the new sexy."

The name of my disease translates directly from the Greek and Latin to "grave weakness."

.*. *.* .*.

When my therapist is back behind her desk, she fills the space between us with charts, and with more diagrams of the human esophagus in various states of distress and relaxation. She handwrites recommendations on jaunty yellow paper, warns me against the use of straws for sipping.

I listen to her, ask questions, nod at appropriate times.

In the window behind her, the hang gliders seem to grow as parallax plays its tricks on their gliding bodies. Their forms become more substantial as they loom closer, cresting on the wind that flows down from the mountain. They swoop close enough that I can see the distinct curves of their muscles against the pale fall sunlight.

I don't look away. I have to admit that they are beautiful.

WHAT MY SELF-RESPECT LOOKS LIKE

Driving home one day, I was stuck behind a slow-going Seattle city bus bearing a large-format ad for a clothing store. The ad featured a man in a blazer being stared at (somewhat ominously, in my opinion) by a woman in a snug and elaborately style-lined dress, oiled legs, and flat-ironed hair. The text of the ad read, "Effort is back in style."

I had to chuckle; dressing myself up the way that she did would take more than effort. For me, it would take a series of minor miracles.

Having muscular weakness means that, on the worst days, holding up a hairdryer simply isn't possible, and that managing to get some mascara on without stabbing myself in the eyeball feels like a CV-worthy achievement. Putting on a dress with the zipper up the back, like the dress in the ad? Not going to happen. Send in the leggings, please.

Unhappily for me, my beloved leggings and yoga pants are current favorite targets of public scorn: everyone wants a say on stretchy pants, including Montana State Senator David Moore, who believes that yoga pants should be illegal to wear in public and has introduced legislation to better achieve his dream of a leggings-free Montana. Then there are the many school districts across the US that have banned girls from wearing stretchy pants to school, ostensibly to shield young boys from the distraction of girls and their bodies. But Emily Dunnagan, principal of one such school in Petaluma, California, dropped the rhetoric about protecting those distractible boys; she was reported by *Huffington Post* as saying that the goal of the ban is simply "... to teach kids to respect themselves."[1]

Ah, self-respect. That was a term I heard quite a bit while I was growing up Christian. At my religious high school, we girls had to kneel and have our skirts measured by a joyless and terrifying administrator. Shorts or anything with spaghetti straps were strictly forbidden, even though it was warm and sweaty California. Piercings were out, too, as were any "countercultural hairstyles," whatever those were.

Our strict dress code was intended, I suppose, to cultivate this nebulous self-respect Dunnagan references, but the result was (at least for me) a cultivation of disrespect for others; I admit that I had, for a long time, dogged standards about not only how I should look, but also about how other women should look. When I was young and relatively healthy, I was so uptight about my personal style that I didn't even own a pair of jeans. My wardrobe was all wool skirts, red lipstick, vintage sweaters, and heels. I looked down my not inconsiderable Germanic nose at women walking around bare-faced and in sweats or yoga pants. *Have a little self-respect*, I thought. *A little dignity*.

I finally got a real education in self-respect after I had major surgery, and my prescribed rehabilitation included walks around the neighborhood. First I was to stumble around for five minutes a day, then ten, then 20. I wasn't prepared for how hard it would be just to stand, much less to get from my door to the driveway and finally to the curb. I was equally unprepared for how difficult it would be to put on clothes—getting into a t-shirt and a pair of yoga pants, and then finally lacing up my sneakers took a laughably long time. The whole process was exhausting enough that I had to lie down as soon as I'd finished dressing.

Before long, I realized I could have one or the other: an exercise-appropriate outfit or my prescribed rehab. *Screw it*, I thought. *I choose walking.*

So that's how I came to be the vision that I was, shuffling slowly thorough my neighborhood in my sunglasses and a pair of pajamas, my unwashed hair sticking up antennae-like as I eventually turned my twenty minutes of walking into 25, then 30. I could hear my younger self tut-tutting in the back of my mind. *You slob*, I could hear her saying. *You can't even stuff yourself into a pair of yoga pants? Show a little self-respect.*

But here's the thing: the me in my mid-thirties, subjecting morning commuters to my daily progress through the streets with my oily face, rogue hair, and tatty pajamas has a whole lot more self-respect than did the me at age 22, with my full face of makeup and body-con outfit; my self-respect no longer hinges on how I look to others.

While it's true that I still feel my best when I'm in a snazzy little outfit, when my eyeliner's perfectly flicked, and when my hair's freshly cut, I've learned that I don't need those things to feel happy with myself. I've learned that other women don't need those things in order for me to respect them, either. And what none of us need? People like Moore and Dunnagan telling us what our self-respect should look like in public.

THE POWER OF DISBELIEF

The summer after I graduated from high school, I went to a backyard barbecue thrown by my new boyfriend. Zach was a talented artist and musician, hip and good looking and cool in every way that I wasn't. We'd been dating for just a few weeks, and this would be my first opportunity to meet his friends. I *really* liked this boy, so my motivation to make a good impression was high. After Zach introduced me around, I did what I often do when I want people to like me: I tried to make myself helpful.

I and my plate of snacks set up next to an improvised court where some of Zach's friends were playing a friendly volleyball game. When the ball bounced out of bounds and rolled in my direction, I chased it down, planning to toss it back to the players. This was my chance, I thought, to make that all-important first impression. *Look, Kelly's nice! She's helpful!* I didn't realize that a different lawn game was taking place right behind me, and I walked straight into the path of an oncoming horseshoe.

When a metal horseshoe travels with some speed and connects with a human skull, the noise it makes is surprisingly like that of a gong. I didn't fully comprehend what had happened—only that something, some incredibly loud and resonant *something*, had felled me. I can't say with certainty whether I blacked out or just lay there on the lawn, stunned, but when I opened my eyes, the faces of all the people I'd met for the first time just minutes before loomed into my field of vision. And then their hands were on me.

They spoke in tongues. They commanded me to be healed. They anointed me *in Jesus's name.* This touching and muttering went on for some minutes. Then they helped me stand and went about the rest of the barbecue. I have a vague recollection of someone handing me a veggie burger.

Today I wonder what kind of person doesn't either call for help or offer somebody a ride to the hospital if she's just sustained a head injury, but their reaction didn't seem off to me at the time. All of us were "Charismatics" (read: Pentecostals) at the time. Any given week, we were more likely to watch an impromptu exorcism in youth group than we were to sing something out of a hymnal. If there wasn't a great deal of hand-raising and weeping and commanding of spirits, it wasn't a real church service. And if you weren't healed of a sickness or an injury after being prayed over, you simply—in a convenient if theologically hazy loophole—didn't have adequate faith.

You just had to try enough. Have faith enough.

I'm no longer part of the church, and I haven't been for years. I'd like to tell you that it's different out here in the rest of the world; I'd like to say that it's better and that people are more likely to give you a hand than lay hands on you, yet I haven't found that to be the case. When you're visibly sick or disabled, everyone, whether friend or stranger, has something for you to put your faith in.

A few years ago, everyone was peddling yoga. *You've really got to try Bikram*, a stranger in Keen sandals would tell me, then talk a great deal about "the breath." After yoga, it was essential oils. In fact, the first time I found myself in the neurology intensive care unit, unable to speak or move, someone helpfully contacted me to suggest that I apply some lavender oils to myself to help me relax, as if I were spending the day at a spa. Today it's the paleo diet—if you're not already gnawing on meat and raw silage, someone will be very happy to tell you the manifold ways in which doing so will not only cure all your medical problems but also bring about world peace at the same time. A natural-healing practitioner told me of her suggested course of edible treatment, "You have to *believe* it'll work."

I recognize that all of these suggestions, from going vegan to taking up pre-dawn calisthenics, come from a well-intentioned place. Those who want to lay hands on people or apply smelly oils to them are, I believe, generally goodhearted. But whatever the impulse, the message I hear is, "If you're still sick, it's your own damn fault. You're not trying hard enough."

Yoga is good exercise for those who can do it, but it's not going to cure a neuromuscular disease. Lavender smells okay, but won't reverse the course of a progressive illness. I have eaten from every diet imaginable, and not a single one does me any more good than the next. And that's okay with me.

In the past few years, I've found incredible power in disbelief. I no longer waste emotional energy scouring my conscience, asking myself whether I'm *really* trying. I no longer feel compelled to down whatever suspicious-looking supplement a distant family member foists on me simply to appear as though I'm exploring every option. When my doctor says a new treatment has a 40% shot at helping, I assume he means 40%, not 100.

Disbelieving that I'll be miraculously healed isn't the same thing as no longer wanting to get well. Instead, it's the understanding that it's okay if I don't. Rather than berate myself over whether I'm doing enough, I've decided to live as though I am enough. I don't know what my life would look like if I were well, but this life—the one I have now—is a pretty good one. It's enough.

SICK GIRL WALKING

Not long after we began exercising together, my husband turned to me and asked, with a pained look, "Is this really something we have to do for the rest of our lives?" I told him that I understood regularity to be part of the whole exercise *thing*, and he actually shuddered.

We've never been too athletic, so it's a mercy for us that the gym we use is populated almost entirely by other people connected to our local Tech Giant. In my experience, software engineers and those of us who love them are more apt to take part in sports whose names include the word "fantasy" than in a session of CrossFit. Most of us heaving ourselves back and forth on the elliptical machines wear baggy, many-years-old t-shirts promoting obsolete software products, and everybody ignores one another as much as possible while we're sweating and breathing heavily with about six inches of space between us. This is the kind of gym for me.

The problem, though, is that everything I need—the women's locker room, the cardio equipment, the bathroom—is upstairs. Up lots and lots of stairs.

I can't really say I'm surprised. After all, the gym is a place that's all *about* physical ability. It's not as though the facility was laid out with the disabled person in mind. It's an assumption of the building's design that, if you're "fit" (a term I hate, by the way) enough to shuffle along on the treadmill or swing some free weights around, you're fit enough to climb a flight of stairs. Yet stairs require a whole different set of motor abilities, and they aren't exactly a friend to many of us with disabilities both visible and invisible. If, for just two examples among many, you have foot drop (trouble lifting up the front half of your foot), or, like me, muscle weakness that makes your knees crumple beneath you at unpredictable intervals, stairs are both slow going and dangerous.

My gym does have a little Elevator of Shame that I'm sure meets the requirements of the Americans with Disabilities Act, but it's a far cry from being a positive experience to ride. Using the clunky thing requires a trip through the mass of humanity swarming the downstairs athletic shop and a long wait while whatever freight task the elevator's also being used for is accomplished. Once upstairs, it spits the rider out somewhere behind a coffee bar (where there's perpetually and inexplicably a man vacuuming the same square foot of space without giving one damn whether anybody can leap out of his way before he trips her).

So stairs it is. On a good day, I'll get a clear shot at the handrail, and I can make my way up, Jell-O knees and all, without incident. On an okay day, I may have to climb, stair by slow stair, behind a toddler who's just learning to walk. (Sometimes my looming behind these kids frightens them. To the little guy who pointed at me and shouted, "Mom, I'm really scared of the lady," my apologies.)

But on a bad day, I end up behind a pair or trio of women—often the same ones, though not always—who stop mid-flight and lean on the handrail for a lengthy confab. The scene is roughly the same every time: I clear my throat to alert these women that someone's waiting behind them. I wait.

Eventually I say, "Excuse me."

The women look at me for a moment, then resume their conversation.

"Excuse me," I say again. "I need to use the handrail."

Once, when I was very lucky, they moved without argument. But most of the time, the women take my request as an invitation to scoff and make icky faces at what I guess they take to be my lazy-cow-ness, and tell me to walk around them.

Sometimes I'll tell them *I can't*, and other times I'll give them a look that would melt steel. Other times I give up, shuffle around them and their overstuffed gym bags, and risk tumbling to the tile floor below because there's honestly a limit to how much confrontation I can handle in one morning. Usually I vow never to take the stairs again.

But then I take the stairs the next time, not because I have a deluded belief I'll get any better at climbing them, but because I hope that one day these women will have some kind of breakthrough of the imagination— that they'll hear me say, "I need to use the handrail," and think, really think, about what I mean. I'm waiting for it to occur to them that, just because someone like me *looks* like she should be able to hoof it up and down a few flights doesn't mean she *is* able. I'm waiting for the day that people think about sharing public space—even this ability-driven, ability-focused space that is the gym—with different kinds of bodies.

FLESH IS FLESH

The late 1990s weren't the most auspicious time to become a vegetarian. Meatless food of any interest hadn't yet entered the American mainstream, so there wasn't much beyond lentils or chunks of naked and jiggling tofu to recommend itself in school cafeterias.

At the same time vegetarianism was beginning to seem less spooky or militant even to devoted meat-eaters; most people knew at least one vegetarian, and they could see that it wasn't part of our daily lives to chain ourselves to the gates of factory farms or engage others in long conversations about "macrobiotics." By 2000, there was even typically a vegetarian item available in any given restaurant, so we could avoid the embarrassment of haggling with waiters over whether the kitchen could maybe just leave the chicken *off* the pasta, thanks. Where was the challenge? The gamesmanship?

Yet it was in that cultural moment, smack between having too few options to eat and having a sea of choices, that I climbed onto the vegetarian bandwagon.

Eating meat had bothered me for a long time, mostly from an aesthetic standpoint. I didn't like the look of it, the feel of it in my mouth. But I'd also developed a private (not wholly articulated or even wholly examined) theory that if I could reduce the suffering that other creatures expended on my part, I'd go some way toward lessening what I saw as my net negative impact on the universe. It was a kind of personal penalty for existing, for taking up mass and energy and resources.

Look, I'm not saying it made sense.

Some years ago I was speaking at a conference in the South, a place where, at least in the mind of this West Coast girl, everyone was supposed to be eating barbecue, and loads of it. After a long day of workshops and talks, we presenters wandered to a nearby Thai restaurant, and I found myself going through the meatless menu with one of the other speakers. As the only two vegetarians in the room—I a sometimes faltering one and she a new member of the fold—we got to talking. I learned she'd given up meat after enduring cancer treatment and what sounded like a brutal double mastectomy. The mere idea of cutting and forking her way into tissue was enough to make her queasy after that. Her illness had given her a heavy-to-carry compassion—a hard-won identification other bodies. Flesh is flesh, after all.

One of the first things I lost when I got sick was the ability to swallow. I would cook the same elaborate, texturally delightful meals I'd always enjoyed, then choke after four or five bites. I'd wait an hour or several for my muscle strength to come back, then eat another four or five bites. Any meal could turn into a day-long gladiatorial battle.

Dining out with friends turned into sitting out with friends. I'd pretend not to be hungry while others ate, even while my stomach growled audibly and I grew dizzy with hunger. I'd go home at the end of the night and pulverize some fruit and powdered protein into a smoothie, or mash some boiled-soft vegetables into a soup thin enough to gag down.

There's only so much blended vegetation a person can drink before she starts thinking about eating something substantial, something toothsome.

I began fantasizing about food while lying in bed at night, trying to sleep while my stomach ached and burned. I dreamed about eating a steak—something I hadn't touched in years. If somebody could put that steak into an unnatural union with some pieces of bacon, I'd applaud. The bizarre culinary acts that Julia Child performed with giant heads of cod on *The French Chef* started to seem like great ideas. The animal suffering that had concerned me for years grew harder to conceptualize. Wasn't starving pound after pound off my dwindling body a kind of animal suffering, too?

During these long nights, I'd tell myself that if the day came when I could eat again—really *eat*—I'd consume everything my greedy teeth could bite. I wouldn't be bothered by ethics or divisions between animal, vegetable, or mineral—bring on the veal and send in the *foie gras*. I didn't care if the fish on my plate had swum free or enjoyed a nice life. In fact (and I'm not proud of this) some part of me almost hoped it suffered. I would eat it and all of its kin into extinction if it meant that I would grow strong as I assimilated their flesh into mine. I would grow larger and larger until my body could accommodate the dark and ravenous pit that had opened inside me. I was owed.

I'm not saying this made sense, either.

Over a period of years, I eventually gained back enough muscle strength to swallow solid food, and I spent many months resembling nothing so much as an actor in a denture fixative commercial delightedly tucking into an ear of corn. My body finally plumped back up to a decent size, and my hair started to grow again. My eyes don't look a jaundiced yellow anymore, and I no longer have much interest in consuming animals beyond a passing whim for a turkey sandwich now and again.

I realize that the more brutal aspects of my inner carnivore were the products of being "hangry" for several years' time. The dark little pit in my heart closed back up. But now I know it's there. I know I'm not among those improved by illness, ennobled by wasting away. I'm in that other camp—the one for those of us who've seen what ugliness we're capable of in all our hunger, all our human need.

YOU HAVE KIDS, RIGHT?

As a woman, you never know when the question is coming—only that it is. You may be having a perfectly innocuous conversation about the traffic, your favorite brand of peanut butter, or even your latest dental work when someone springs it on you: "You have kids, right?"

A couple of years ago, while I was representing the literary journal I co-edit at a small but hopping book expo in Seattle, an aspiring writer parked himself in front of my table and began to regale me with a lengthy description of a poem, probably one he'd written himself. I confess that, after a while, I wasn't really listening—I was amusing myself with the fact that his voice sounded almost identical to David Lynch's, and I was wondering whether I could somehow direct the conversation toward the forthcoming *Twin Peaks* reboot for my own amusement. That's when he asked, apropos nothing, if I had kids. I replied that I did not.

"Oh, you'd never understand the poem, then," he told me.

My tolerance for men patronizing me is notably low, so I turned to my co-publisher and said, about as loudly as possible, "Joe, you hear that? I can't understand poetry because I don't have children!"

A few people turned our direction and chuckled, and poor Joe looked mortified, but the man who was not David Lynch didn't seem to recognize that I was making fun of him. He carried on, probably explaining how his perceptual powers had been raised by causing some poor woman to birth his offspring. I was too busy fantasizing about kicking his teeth in to pay further attention. He finally moved on to another table—presumably to find somebody whose poetry comprehension had been elevated through childbirth—and I tried to forget about the incident, but it kept gnawing at me for the rest of the day.

I'm a happily childless person, so if even I wanted to relieve the man who wasn't David Lynch of his full set of teeth, I can't imagine how a woman dealing with infertility must feel when she hears the same kinds of insensitive comments. I have never longed for a baby, and I haven't felt my life to be incomplete for the lack of one. I'm everybody's auntie and nobody's mom, and take great pleasure in spoiling the children in my life before sending them home to their parents. But I'm fully aware that these facts are unimaginable to some, and that they make me, in these people's eyes, something less than an actual woman.

I'm also aware of the fact that, even if I wanted a child, it isn't the best idea to give birth to one. The drugs that keep me above ground are toxic—so toxic, in fact, that they carry black box warnings so scary that my doctor asked me three times while writing the prescription whether I was *sure* that I *never* wanted kids. Even if there existed a magical, cellular-level eraser that could scrub all the poison from my body, any baby I carried would still have a one in five shot at having the same disease that I do, but at such an amplified severity that he or she would likely die not long after birth. Death on arrival doesn't seem like a good gamble.

I'm not a person who can't imagine loving a child who was anything less than the picture of health, or of whom I couldn't brag to other parents about various measurement percentiles (it seems to me, as an outside observer, that parenting an infant has a great deal to do with ranking babies against one another in some kind of percentile-related horserace). This may be my own bias, but I believe we sick people are as capable of meaningful living—and as capable of loving and being loved—as anybody.

But just as there are people like the man who wasn't David Lynch who can't imagine a childless woman, there are also legions of people who can't imagine having a sick kid. We all know them. We've heard expecting parents say, "I don't care if it's a boy or a girl, just as long as it's healthy." Then they look particularly solemn while stroking their bellies. We all know how we're supposed to interpret their statements—we're meant to hear it as magnanimity and a desire not to see their offspring suffer. But we who are sick understand intuitively that we are, in these people's minds, the worst possible outcome. We are the spooky unknown. We embody others' darkest fears. Sometimes we are less, in their eyes, than full people.

So here I am: a great failure of modern womanhood. The person who hasn't fulfilled—and won't ever fulfill—her biological endgame. A woman whose own biology has gotten away from her.

From this other side of great chasm of human progress, I can tell you that being the worst possible outcome—the scary, not-quite-real woman—isn't all that bad. In fact, my life is downright ordinary and satisfying. I have meaningful relationships with the people in my life—that includes adults *and* children. I find fulfillment in my work. I have my little family of two. I enjoy a vivid imaginative life.

Hell, I even understand poetry.

THE SMELL OF TEMPERED GLASS

Open the nearest paperback, crack it open, and take a good, deep whiff. Nice, right? I'm not going to tell you how many dust mites and fruiting bodies you probably just hoovered into your sinus cavity. That would ruin whatever enjoyment you just got out of that dose of musty old book smell. It's one of those weird pleasures—like packed earth after rain—that a lot of people just can't get enough of.

I used to feel the same way about that smell. I'm about as big a book lover as you could possibly meet; for a time, I made a living as an editor at a British publishing company, I run a literary magazine, and have, so far, published two books of my own (you're looking at one of them right now). When I moved to England, the bulk of what I brought with me was books—and those were only the books I thought I would *desperately need*. If you told me that the afterlife would involve being cryogenically suspended in a tank with the text of books projected on a gel medium that I could read for eternity, I'd be thrilled. You get the idea—my life revolves around the written word.

Yet those piles of hardcovers and dog-eared paperbacks heaped around my home are getting dustier and funkier all the time; a fat copy of Marlon James's *A Brief History of Seven Killings* has lived on my nightstand for the better part of a year now, but every time I settle in for a long read, I make it through about four paragraphs at best. I lay the book back down on the table beside me, wait a few days or weeks, then start the effort again, but I never get far. I can't make out the words.

Like most people who have myasthenia gravis, I often experience double vision. The outlines of objects in my view may be slightly blurred, or I may see two distinct images of the same thing. There's nothing wrong with my eyes themselves, but rather with what holds them in place; my muscles are too weak to keep my vision in focus. Even on days when I don't see double, one or the other of my eyes may droop or even close entirely. Trying to read tiny print on pulp paper can feel like watching a silent film through a keyhole—I can see only by glimpses and flickers, floating images of black-on-white.

As you might imagine, my eyes have had an impact on the way I go about my editing and writing life. Some people like me resort to double-sided tape or even to surgical stitches to hold their eyelids up and help them see, but neither seems like a particularly appealing solution to me. Instead, I manage my day job with the help of a massive computer monitor—the sort of thing on which a NASA engineer could no doubt plot a Mars mission in vivid detail—on which I amplify each document I'm working on by orders of magnitude. A colleague likes to joke that he can tell which shared documents I've looked at lately because they're all scaled to 400%. While that may be an exaggeration, it's only a slight one.

We get by, my giant documents and I, with our towering letters floating against the white page. Yet at each day's end, when all I want is to read a good novel for the pure pleasure of it, the text of the books stacked in my To Be Read pile is sometimes as inaccessible to me as cuneiform.

Enter the greatest gift that technology has given to book lovers: the e-reader. As soon as I tried ebooks in lieu of paperbacks, I was hooked: I could adjust the size of the text to my giant specifications, change the font to something easier to track, and play with the brightness level on the screen until I found what was best for my tricky little muscles. As much as I always enjoyed the tactile experience of a paper book, I wouldn't hesitate to trade my entire collection of physical books in for digital versions; ebooks have given reading back to me. If being able to read again means learning to love the smell of tempered glass, then I'm game.

But ebooks have given me something else: plenty of belittling by strangers. To talk openly with other bookish folks about my love of ebooks is practically to wear a sign saying, "I would like to hear a public referendum on why my choices are terrible and damaging to the publishing industry." Even when I explain in clear terms that I can't always see the print in hard copy, people have told me that I'm just not reading "real" books, and that I'm part of some sort of global problem with low attention spans and so-called "addictions" to tech. I don't even bother with any "The Future of Publishing" talks at writers' conferences anymore—they're inevitably panels of New Yorkers dressed in funeral black and muttering that "we just don't know what's going to happen with all these ebooks."

Even online media outlets—ironically, given their digital DNA—get into ebook-related scolding with flimsy studies and convenient theories: "Hard copy books are just more pleasant to read," *The Washington Post* wants us to know.[2] And, of course, we can't get away from that all-important feature of smell in the appreciation of literature: physical books "look and smell good," according to *CBS News.*[3] (Thanks for those tips, journalists.)

What's behind this anti-ebook snobbery, anyway? And why are people spilling so much ink in defense of hard copy when ebooks (not to mention many other technologies, such as screen readers) have made reading accessible again for a number of people who—like me—would otherwise be shut out from contemporary literature?

I suppose there's the usual pettiness involved: it's the same impulse that makes us battle it out over the right way to squeeze a tube of toothpaste or make sweeping judgments over whether leggings can be worn as pants. Yet I think there's something else—something more sinister—at work: the assumption that there's a default mode of living, and that that mode is firmly centered on what the "normal" person is capable of doing.

That assumption's there in the way we regard the person who circles the lot so that she can park her car nearest to the door *(Can't she walk a few extra feet?)*. It's there in the side-eye we cast at the man riding a scooter in the grocery store, silently sizing him up *(He's probably just lazy)*. It's there in the perky little posters on elevator doors encouraging us to take the stairs instead *(It's healthy!)*.

It's there, too, in the language often used in criticizing others. How often do we read that someone is "blind" to facts, "deaf" to tone, "lame" in behavior, "crippled" by fear, or "paralyzed" by doubt? Even our metaphors are steeped in the ridicule of people who don't fit an entrenched view of normality.

And that, friends, is *ableism:* the notion that the able body is the right body, and that the disabled body is an aberration. It's the view that life in a disabled body isn't simply a different kind of life, but that it's a lesser one.

To some people, ableism doesn't seem like that big of a problem; at times, when I've pointed out rude language or hurtful actions, I've been asked whether I'm not just looking for something to be offended by, as though offense were a nice side-table I've been searching for to complement my sofa. How could a few ugly looks or careless remarks really impact anybody's life, people want to know.

To ask such questions, though, is to approach the problem from the wrong end entirely. Rude language and antisocial behavior are ableism's mildewy stink—not the worst of the decay itself. At the deep and rotting core, the idea that able bodies are better bodies has consequences that are as tangible as they are serious. Consider the US government's allowance of a sub-minimum wage for disabled workers[4] (contributing, unsurprisingly, to an astronomical rate of poverty among the disabled), the withholding of appropriate medical treatment from people considered unworthy of expensive care (as when Amelia Rivera, a three-year-old, was denied a medically appropriate kidney transplant because of her Wolf-Hirschhorn syndrome[5]), and even state-sanctioned murder (as when 12-year-old Tracy Latimer, who had cerebral palsy, was murdered by her overwhelmed father, Robert Latimer, who pumped exhaust into the cab of his Chevy truck and looked on as Tracy died of carbon monoxide poisoning. Canadian courts exempted Robert from typical sentencing guidelines because the crime, as they viewed it, was committed for "caring and altruistic reasons"[6]).

So, no. Somebody making snide remarks about why I shouldn't be reading ebooks—even when I've made it clear that those books are pretty much all I've got—isn't going to kill me. But the attitude that makes those remarks seem okay? That attitude *does* kill.

None of this is to say that anyone should give up their stinky old books. I hope that people enjoy them, sniffing those old bindings until they're sneezing with glee. But I also hope that they'll think twice before putting down those who get the same thrill from tempered glass.

I WAS ONCE THE WRITER KELLY DAVIO

I'm pretty good at falling. Over the past few years of living with myasthenia gravis, I've learned how to come down on the flats of my hands without jamming my wrists, and even if my knees bruise, I can always wear something that covers the worst of the marks so I don't look like the victim of some kind of alarming knee-related crime.

I've had a lot of time to work on my form. At times, my tumbles were such a part of daily life that my husband even came up with an Olympic-style system for rating my falls. He'd hear a thump as I hit the floor in some far corner of our home, then come in to help me up, but only after giving me a mostly arbitrary score of *seven* or *eight-point-five* after assessing how I'd stuck my landing. If that sounds cold, it wasn't. We found it funny; the sicker I got, the more we both needed a good laugh.

There came a point when I couldn't get between pieces of furniture in my house without taking a spill, and no matter how practiced I was at landing well, I was starting to feel the effects of daily falls—an ache here, an unhappily pulled muscle there. At my worst, when I needed to get farther than five or six feet at a time in a public place—say, from a far end of a parking lot to a building—I'd end up hanging off my husband's arm like a pet sloth.

Finally I had to admit I needed a cane; there were times when I had no shoulder to hang from, and I needed a better strategy than hoping I'd magically stay upright every moment I was alone.

So, I did it: I ordered myself a green paisley cane. Fifteen bucks, two days, and some free Prime shipping later, and I was in business.

I loved my new cane. I could stand up more quickly, walk across a parking lot without beefing it in front of an oncoming SUV, and get across tricky rooms without having to hold on to walls like a creeping insect. My life was monumentally improved.

Who knew a fifteen-dollar piece of aluminum could do all that?

. *.* *.*

Some months after I started clacking along on my spiffy new assistive device, I attended the AWP—or Association of Writers and Writing Programs—conference in Seattle: it was a big, teeming mass of creative writers, many of whom I'd known professionally for years. Before entering the vast conference center, I gave myself an unconvincing little parking lot pep talk: *Maybe nobody will notice you're sick this year! It'll be fine!* Heaving myself out of the car with my cane, I felt like a grade school kid worrying about what the schoolyard bullies would say about her Coke-bottle glasses.

Yet I was a grown woman, amid a sea of other grown people. Surely nobody would point out what was so obviously embarrassing to me.

I shuffled into the conference hall, repeating *it'll be fine* in the back of my brain while I missed session after session; there was no way I could move quickly enough through swarming crowds to make my way between distant points of the building. So I stopped to chat with people.

There was a great deal of noticeable name-tag scanning when I greeted folks I'd known for years but who didn't recognize me with those drugs that aged me, hair that had thinned considerably, face puffed up with steroids, and my body thirty pounds lighter than it should've been. I got tired of saying a boisterous hello to people who either couldn't recognize this version of me or wanted to know, "What happened to you?" Exhausted and demoralized, I ducked into a panel discussion—one where, mercifully, there was somewhere to sit.

One of the speakers on the panel was talking about the importance of believability in fiction, and led into a point with, "as the writer Kelly Davio said ..." I listened with horror as she repeated what I expected to be some poorly considered remark I'd made on Twitter. The look on my face probably resembled that of a wombat being asked to do calculus.

Mercifully, the panelist wasn't calling me out, but actually illustrating a point she was making. To my great surprise, I'd actually been trotted out as some kind of authority. When I left the talk twenty or so minutes later, I felt a hell of a lot better about myself. I was, after all, The Writer Kelly Davio. I had been quoted!

With this new feeling that I was *somebody*—despite being an unrecognizable, cane-hobbling shade of myself—I ventured out into the chaos of people in the book fair halls and tried being social again.

It was while shuffling through the corridors with my renewed sense of confidence that I felt the fist in my back. A man walking behind me had, for no reason I can imagine, punched me between the shoulder blades.

I flew forward. I came down, knees cracking hard on the concrete floor, trying to fall so that I wouldn't injure myself, but failing in the brute surprise of it all.

As the meat of my hands swelled up from the impact, my mind played catch-up with the reality of my body on the ground. I tried to sort out what had just happened—this had to be some kind of freak accident, didn't it? But what kind of accident involves punching someone? Who goes around swinging balled-up fists in a crowded room to begin with?

I looked up to see the man who had just hit me laughing as he loomed above me in his ugly red sweatshirt. It didn't seem like the way a person behaves after a freak accident.

I waited for any one of the scores of people standing around and gawking to offer me some help. Any moment, I thought, someone would confront this man who'd just clocked me in the middle of a packed convention center. Of course one of these hundreds of other writers would offer to help me stand up, or even simply ask if I was okay.

But each of the people who'd just watched a strange man hit me turned back to their business, and the crowd bustled on as though I wasn't there.

I watched their pretty shoes step past me as I crawled, on hands and knees, to reach my cane. I watched them maneuver around my body as I scooped up my absurd little conference tote bag and its ridiculous bookmarks and pens and submission guidelines that had spilled out all over the floor. I watched dozens of people pass and pretend not to notice as the man who'd just punched me reached down and picked me up off the floor, pressing himself against my back in a way that made me want to vomit or shower or both.

This is the part of the story when I am supposed to rise up from the ground like some kind of avenging spirit. It would make for a good scene if I'd dragged myself up by a festooned tablecloth on one of the trade show stalls—perhaps taking half of an MFA program's table display with me—and let the man have it. It might be even better if I'd let the pamphlets and poetry collections and mailing list sign-up sheets fly around me as I lashed out at him, wielding my aluminum cane like a weapon (though of course I wouldn't *hit* him. I'm not a violent jerk, after all).

Yet that's not what happened.

This is the part of the story when I gathered my things with as much dignity as I could scrape together and walked straight ahead. A man who'd apparently been watching my clobbering unfold from his table a few feet away asked if I'd be interested in purchasing a year-long subscription to his publication. I politely declined. I'm not sure that he deserved my politeness.

This is the part of the story when I found the women's bathroom, shut myself in a stall, and cried.

What a disappointment: a 30-year-old woman sniveling in the restroom like a humiliated child. I know what's expected of sick and disabled people, and this wasn't it. We're to be inspirational, never to break the illusion of perfect equanimity, and—above all—to accept unacceptable circumstances without making a fuss.

Yet if I broke an unspoken social code, so did the mass of people who stood around and gaped at me that day. It would have been just as good a scene, after all, had any of my fellow writers asked if I needed assistance, confronted the man who'd hit me, offered to call security, helped me to a safe location, or even just smiled at me humanely.

This isn't a story about human kindness any more than it's a story about fortitude.

This is the story of how I learned I wasn't The Writer Kelly Davio any longer. I wasn't someone to quote—I was *something* to walk over. And why? What I'd thought had made me awkwardly noticeable had made me, in fact, invisible.

Who knew a fifteen-dollar piece of aluminum could do all that?

II. THE FOUR WHITE WALLS

FALL RISK

I dislike him from the start, the nursing assistant assigned to me. The whiteboard across the room says that his name is Arman, or Arthur. Maybe it's even Arnold—my vision is hazy, and I can't make out what's written in light green marker.

I've just graduated five floors up to the neurology ward from the intensive care unit, a vertical progression that means I'm getting better. Better enough that I don't need an ICU nurse presiding over my bed full-time, at least, and enough that I'm allowed the comfort of the pink, flannel pajama bottoms my husband has retrieved from my drawer at home. I'm still in my hospital gown, but at least I'm warmer now, and covered.

For the next few days, I'll be poked at and medicated by a series of nurses who all seem to be named Kathy, a different one manifesting every 12-hour shift. Their nursing assistants will help me stand for long enough to stretch my legs against the threat of blood clots.

I plan to wait out Arman's shift before I ask for anything—he makes me nervous, standing closer to me than necessary while Kathy the First shines a flashlight in my eyes, peers down into my pupils, and asks if I know where I am.

I don't immediately grasp that she's administering a test. "I'm pretty sure I'm in the hospital."

"I mean *which* hospital."

When I catch on to the fact that she's grading my answers, writing them down and scoring them against some kind of cognitive rubric, I try to do better. I tell her which hospital. I even add the room number, though forming each word takes energy I don't have.

She asks for today's date. I tell her I have no idea. I lost track of time in the ICU, where the lights never go off—no day or night, artificial or otherwise. I haven't been allowed to sip water, much less eat food, so I can tell nothing by the hunger pangs in my belly. I don't have the strength to explain any of this to Kathy.

Arman is standing so close that I can smell his body. I'm fairly sure I've

29

showered more recently than he has, and I've been in the hospital for days. He stares down at me while I answer Kathy's questions.

She asks if I at least know what year it is, and I tell her.

When she's satisfied with my answers and turns to her medicine cart for a syringe of morphine to disgorge into one of my many I.V. lines, I add that Barack Obama is the President of the United States. Kathy smiles. But Arman, still close—too close—laughs. He laughs as though he's never heard such wit. He grabs me beneath the arms and shifts me in bed, though I don't need shifting. His breath is sour in my face.

Strange men have had their hands on me for days.

It started with a nurse whose name I never caught, the one who settled me in for a four-day infusion of other people's blood plasma: the pooled immunoglobulin of fifty-thousand other people, to be more specific. I tried not to watch as he prodded at the blue veins in my arm, looking for a nice, fat vessel. The idea of strangers' bodily fluids dripping into my bloodstream didn't sit well with me, the needle-phobe, the faint-hearted, the squeamish. But with my own immune system gone rogue and attacking my nervous system, I needed to borrow someone else's functional blood, someone else's correct set of antibodies.

In the end I was right to be nervous about the treatment. The first day's infusion seemed to go smoothly enough, and was at least over in time for me to head home for a night's sleep before the next round. But by two in the morning, I was immobile on the floor of my bedroom, prostrated by a case of meningitis—a swelling in the brain and spinal cord—induced by donor plasma.

I couldn't speak. I couldn't open my left eye. I couldn't stand. My husband half-walked, half-dragged me from house to car and car to emergency room. He scribbled my name on documents I couldn't hold a pen to sign. I remember hitting the emergency room floor, gagging from the pain of my brain trying to break through my skull.

The second man's disembodied hands shucked my clothes off and draped my naked chest with a gown. I heard the voice of what I assumed to be a doctor say "brain bleed" to my husband where they stood in the doorway. It occurred to me that I might die. I thought that dying would be alright if it stopped the hammering inside my brain.

I couldn't make out the face of the third man through my barely opened right eye. But I could see the fuzzy green of an old tattoo on his wrist as he slapped at my arm, then gouged into the ditch of my elbow with a needle. Finally a burn of Dilaudid. Then another. Then morphine, morphine, morphine. The edges of my body grew hazy, the narcotics blurring the line between my skin an the cold air of the emergency room.

The fourth man heaved me onto a gurney and wheeled me away. The metallic rattle over the linoleum floor sounded like a jet engine at close range. I could barely hear over the roar when he asked me if I could be pregnant as he placed me inside a CT machine that would scan my brain, looking ruptured blood vessels.

Paramedics arrived, and a fifth man bundled me to a stretcher, said something about a transfer. I remember the jostle of the ambulance's interior, the clanking of metal inside its boxy carriage. The drugs began to work on my mind if not fully on my pain; the EMT's face shifted as he watched me, his black hair sprouting rodent ears, his face growing a long muzzle. To my eyes, he had become a rabbit, burrowing into the gray pulp of my brain.

The sixth man was the ICU neurologist who grabbed my head and tried to shove it to my breastbone to see if my neck would move around my swollen spinal cord. It wouldn't. I remember opening my mouth and trying to scream. After that, a blackness.

The seventh man was the ICU nurse who would tend me around the clock until I could speak, open my eyes, ask for more pain medication. He was clumsy, knocking into me as he maneuvered around the medical equipment packed tightly into the room. He was the first one whom I actually liked—he reminded me of someone I'd have met in a required course in college—some earnest student not entirely adequate to the task of interpreting the textbook, but raising his hand often to ask permutations of the same question. I took comfort in the way he turned his eyes away and made distracting, one-sided conversation when he lifted me to dislodge the EMT's sheet from under my body. I appreciated the illusion of dignity.

Once Kathy the First leaves, I send my husband home to take a long nap and to feed the cat. In a lengthy, fumbling process that takes all the coordination I have, I put in my ear buds and listen to old Elliott Smith albums on my phone. I need the distraction from the incessant clack of my I.V. and from the every-fifteen-minute puff and growl of the blood pressure monitor. The quiet, acoustic strumming—no drums—is all my swollen brain can handle. Maybe it's the morphine draining into my left arm, but "Needle in the Hay" begins to seem like a masterwork of American songwriting.

I must manage to sleep, because the album is over before I've heard half of it, and the angle of sun in the room has shifted. I eye the bathroom a few feet from my bed, and strategize how I might maneuver my I.V. pole all that infinite distance.

On the door to my room is a laminated sign that reads *Fall Risk*. A decorative pattern of red and blue stars gives the placard a patriotic flavor. The sign means that I'm not allowed to stand up on my own, to shuffle to the bathroom, to accommodate my own needs without someone there to heave me up and down, but I'm tired of asking for—and tired of getting—strangers' help.

I get as far as loosening the Velcro on the wheezing, pneumatic compression socks bound to my calves. It's exhausting, and I'm dizzy by the time I'm done. At the change in blood pressure, my brain protests, nerves exploding in a white heat. I give up and press the call button.

It's not a Kathy who comes to help me, but Arman. My voice isn't much better than a whisper when I ask to be walked to the bathroom, and so he leans his head close—too close—to hear me.

When I've made myself understood, he retrieves a black nylon belt from a far corner of the room. It looks like an apparatus meant for moving a piano or an overstuffed sofa. He cinches it around my waist and hauls me to my feet, my arms flapping loose beside me. He shuffles me forward and drags my IV pole beside him. On my leash, I feel as though I'm an elderly dog being taken for a too-fast walk. He takes four steps. I take ten. We make it to the bathroom, and Arman opens the door, clanking my IV pole inside. I say, "Thanks," and wait for him to leave.

Arman doesn't move. "Here, I'll help you," he says.

I don't know what he means. I've made it here already. "I'm fine."

He reaches for my pink pajama bottoms and yanks them down.

"No!" I try to grab my clothes back and cover my naked thighs, but I move as though I'm underwater. My arms won't follow what I ask of them. I say, "Stop." I want my voice to be loud and assertive, but it comes out quiet and slurred. The green bathroom tile swims in front of me in a flicker of overhead lighting, and I think my eyes might rupture.

I repeat the word "stop" over and over until he leaves. Finally the door clanks shut behind him.

I curse ice chips and I curse the IV fluids and I curse the fact that I have kidneys and that they've had to do something with all this accumulated water. I curse the fact that I have a body in the first place.

I hold the metal rail on the wall and lower myself to the cold, sterile seat. Someone is striking an anvil in my brain.

The door peels open.

Arman leans in. He stares at my nakedness until I am finished.

The first lesson of the hospital is that the body belongs to everyone assigned to its care. I am given a flimsy gown and will wear that gown. I am not allowed to eat, though my stomach is roiling after days without a bite of food. Anyone who comes into my room is allowed to touch me, to reach a hand down my gown and root around with a stethoscope, to shove at my head to see if my neck will move. It still won't. Medical students look at me like I'm a colorful bacterial culture in a petri dish as their attending physician talks about my case.

The body is a public place. My own bloodstream, still plump with thousands of strangers' DNA, reminds me of this fact with every skull-splitting heartbeat.

By the time Arman unbelts me and releases me back into the white of my hospital bed, I think my head may be breaking apart, splintering from the inside. As Arman leaves the room, I realize I can barely care about him now. His fumbling hands at my clothing, his eyes on my bare body—all of his slimy attentions pale beside the volcanic urgency of what's happening inside my skull.

If there is a gift in pain, it is that pain is all-consuming; I have no objective but to make it stop. The gift of pain is also its danger. Miles below my consciousness, I know I should be afraid, or angry. But right now I cannot bring myself to care.

Across the ward, a speaker honks out a digitized rendition of "Mary Had a Little Lamb." The tune starts and stops, starts and stops. When an orderly comes into the room, I ask, "What's with the song?"

"Bed alarm," he tells me. A woman across the ward has tended to wander. They've belted her down, but she still manages to break loose and move about without permission. She's another Fall Risk.

I think about Arman strapping her to her bed, her body resisting. I think about him laughing at her with his face too close to hers. I think about him belting me down, his hands on my body where I don't want them but can't protest.

All along the hall, *EXIT* signs glow a hazy red, a red that says, *Stop*. A red that says, *You're not going anywhere*.

JAMES BROWN AND I GO TO THE LAB

In the past year or two of medical treatment, I've learned that it's possible to get used to any number of things I would've previously placed on a spectrum of "I would prefer not to" all the way to "over my dead body." Tolerating such things has nothing to do with personal strength or intestinal fortitude—it's simply a matter of my internal give-a-damn meter no longer going up very high in the face of increasingly bizarre requests:

"We'd like to place some electrified needles in your muscles and see what happens." *Um.*

"We'd also like to infuse your bloodstream with the plasma of roughly fifty thousand other people." *Uh, okay?*

"Also, please take this chemo drug every day for the rest of your life." *Fine. Whatever.*

Despite my best efforts, there are also those demands that I can't get used to. Namely I can't get myself to tolerate a simple blood draw without high drama; the moment a phlebotomist comes walking toward me with gloved hands and a needle, I hyperventilate. I turn a disconcerting shade of green, sometimes cry a little, then pass out like a fainting goat.

My freak-out-and-pass-out routine was embarrassing enough even back in those healthier days when I only needed blood taken with routine physicals. But now that I and my "bad," hard-to-find veins need our blood counts monitored once each week, I can't afford for every trip to the lab to become an hour-long production in which I'm going to fall on the floor, knock my head, cry my eyeliner off, and leave drenched in sweat.

One summer, after a particularly unpleasant lab incident—an occasion on which I blacked out twice while the phlebotomist probed vein after vein and still couldn't "find anything"—I asked friends, strangers, and anybody who'd engage me on the subject how they manage to stay conscious and maintain a little personal dignity while being jabbed with needles.

There were the useless suggestions, such as "Don't watch" while foreign objects puncture your tender little arm flab (trust me: not looking doesn't help), but there were novel ones as well: drink a lot of salty soup to jack up your blood pressure. Suck down a ton of juice. Stay warm—even hot. Get some exercise. Listen to something peppy. Visualize a kitten.

I took everyone's suggestions, and because I didn't know which one might actually help, I took them all at once and with singular devotion. I downed a pint and a half of miso soup and another pint or so of orange juice. I put on my winter mittens and a sweatshirt even though it was 90 degrees outside in mid July. I listened to James Brown encouraging me to turn it loose, or to engage in the separate but related activities of driving my funky soul and getting on the scene. I did some jumping jacks in the parking lot. I imagined cats—several, just to be safe. And when the phlebotomist took my blood, for the first time in years, I neither cried nor fainted. It would be hard to have felt more proud had I just been handed a lifetime achievement award.

So when the lab phoned the next day to say that they'd lost the several vials they'd just taken (though how a facility specializing in the collection of human blood misplaces said blood is beyond me), I was not amused. At least I had my routine now—it may have been elaborate, but I felt that it was repeatable. James Brown and I would be okay.

I gobbled more miso soup. I drank more juice. I drove my funky soul back to the lab, then I got on up in the parking lot (to the great interest of the HVAC technicians outside) while wearing my mittens and picturing cats. Inside the lab, I rolled up my sleeves, presented my arms, and let the phlebotomist get to work. Twenty minutes later, she was still at work, still harpooning for a vein. When a second phlebotomist came over and began stabbing at my other arm, I couldn't hold it together—I burst into my usual snotty tears and fainted.

It's several months and many blood draws later, and I've given up on the idea of ever having a smooth, drama-free visit to the lab. I've had to make peace with the way the technicians say, "Oh, *Kelly's* here," when I sign in while wearing my mittens. But I've decided that this fainting routine is okay. It's never going to be pleasant to wake up in a sweaty heap, but it serves as a reminder to me that I am still a part of this body, not a ride-along mind in a meat jalopy.

The things we sick people are willing to do to get well—or simply not get any worse—can sometimes make us feel that our bodies are old junkers we lug around and routinely drag into the shop for tune-ups. They are separate from the *real* us. They are different. Lesser. Removed from who we are as thinking, emoting people.

Yet it's me, the person, who's scared bloodless by those approaching needles. It's me, the person, who—like it or not—has the emotional reaction that leads to the physical fallout. For once, it's me, the person, who's in some way in control. And the fact that my mind and body aren't ready to part just yet? I'll take it as good news.

ON A SCALE OF ONE TO TEN

The health care system I've used for some years prides itself in displaying laminated pain scale cards in each of its offices. Whether I'm in the physical therapist's room with its suspicious-looking cords and pulleys or in my neurologist's office being knocked upon with a hammer, everybody wants me to consult the pain scale and identify my discomfort by a number.

The card features a range of cartoons helpfully arranged in order of misery. From left to right, the little numbered faces range from chipper (indicated by perky eyebrows) to suffering grievously (suggested by what are either tears or cheek goiters.)

I make a dutiful attempt to pick something appropriate, but the only intervals on the scale that make sense to me are zero ("Totally fine, nothing to see here!") and ten ("I welcome the sweet embrace of death."). The rest of the rankings are hazy to me, partly because they move by multiples of two, and the jumps between facial expressions seem a little drastic; somewhere between 6 and 8, the smiley face looks as though it's been the victim of a terrible crime. Whatever happens to a person at 7 or 7.5, I don't want to know about it.

Even when trying my best, I'm terrible at sorting out what's what on the scale. Is a migraine a 4 or a 5? Is a dislocated rib a 6 or a 7? Experience tells me to just aim for something low unless I want a disbelieving look or a furtive note written in my chart. However I feel, I just call it a 3.

As if the pain scale didn't offer enough bodily arithmetic, the more complicated I've become medically, the more incomprehensible the calculations I'm asked to do. When assessing my candidacy for a surgical intervention some time ago, the head of the department at the hospital asked me to tell him by what percentage I'd been debilitated by my neurological disease.

"What percentage?" I had prepared myself for all kinds of possible outcomes in this consultation. I was ready for anything from his brushing me off to telling me that I'd need one of the more gross and undesirable procedures for which he's famous among his peers. One thing I hadn't prepared for was performing quality-of-life math on the spot. I didn't know how to put a number to the way I lived, or to the extent to which I'd adapted, year after year, to a new and inadequate set of circumstances. "I have no idea."

He assured me that he just wanted an estimate.

At this point, I was emotionally exhausted, and I was frustrated. As I often do when frustrated, I said whatever came to mind.

"I haven't been able to chew a salad for three years. I can't teach for the duration of a whole class anymore. I can't walk anywhere without falling. I stop breathing sometimes. You tell me what percentage that is."

He stopped typing away at his computer, swiveled around in his chair to look at me, and smoothed out his tie. "I think you answered my question."

He performed my surgery three months later.

For a time, I assumed that my reluctance to get behind assigning numeric values to my life had something to do with what the mathematician John Allen Paulus called "innumeracy," or the "mathematical analogue of functional illiteracy." As a teenager, I bought wholeheartedly into what I heard so often: girls aren't good at math (why anybody was telling perfectly capable girls that they were inherently deficient in any academic subject is a topic for another day), and I expected very little of myself when it came to quantifying the world. I freely admit that I am among the people whom Paulus says "readily understand narrative particulars, but strongly resist impersonal generalities."[7]

I concluded that it was my own, innumerate fault, this perplexity with the pain chart and my befuddlement with the business of assigning percentages to disability. I took it as a personal failure that I couldn't grasp the *impersonal generalities* folded up inside my experience. What did it matter to the doctor, after all, whether I could chew a salad? Why would he care how long I could lecture to a class before I couldn't breathe anymore? It had nothing to do with him or with the cost/benefit analysis of cutting me open.

Have I been treating my personal experience as too, well, *personal*? Is it time to get onboard with those impersonal generalities? Maybe. But I've found myself incapable of doing so. And it's not, I've decided, that I've got such an extreme case of innumeracy that I can't deal with reality. Instead, I've realized that the medical world's insistence on dealing with patients by impersonal numbers is quite convenient when it comes to treating us as problems, not as people.

This fact came home to me while I was going through the details of the health insurance I'd be obliged to use when I moved to the United Kingdom from Seattle. Here are a few of the insurer's impersonal numbers: zero (the amount of benefit a patient is allowed for incurable illnesses, such as the one I've got), and five (the number of years I'd have to be medication-free before the company would even think about offering me care). Back in the US, I was already familiar with six (hundred dollars per month for a single drug). I knew also about 25 (thousand dollars for the single dose of donor plasma that's a standby of treatment for patients like me). These numbers are not impersonal. They are the equivalent of being told to take a running jump off a cliff. They are numbers that hurt.

I think I've had enough of impersonal generalities when it comes to my body. I'm not going to be able to convince insurers that my life is worth preserving, of course, but I am going to start where I can, with my private war against the pain scale. In this month's bevy of appointments, I'm foregoing the little faces on the chart. "Do you mind if we don't do the numbers?" I plan to ask. "Let me tell you what it feels like."

THE SERVICE OF LESSER GODS

In my youth, it wasn't uncommon to see people collapse. Whole groups of them might go at once in an invisible sea swell that washed over five or ten people at a time.

I'd stand in my brown upholstered church pew, shifting from foot to foot, watching as the adults around me dropped to the floor or into the arms of the church elders. On the platform at the front of the church, a keyboardist would quietly play chords on an old Yamaha while the minister held up one arm, or maybe both, over the crowd. He'd mutter over the bodies on the floor in what sounded like a language from some distant star.

Even if this scene wasn't unusual, it was always strange. The church members called this phenomenon "being slain in the spirit," a term I could never quite understand. I'd been hearing since I was in Sunday school that God wanted to give us life. So what did he want with slaying us?

From time to time, other children would walk forward to the church altar and take their turns at being slain—letting the minister push the heel of his hand down on their foreheads until they swooned over and hit the rough carpet. But I stayed put. I wanted nothing to do with being killed, even by God himself.

I waited in the surgeon's consultation room through the afternoon, the unexpected March sunlight streaking through the window and warming my back to a sweat.

I'd dressed well, or at least tried. Years of medical appointments had taught me to neaten up for doctors. I wanted to look like a person who was doing her best—a person who hoped that, in turn, the surgeon would do *his* best. Even if I'd wanted to throw on a comforting t-shirt or my "feel-better sweater" and track pants, the doctor would certainly come in wearing his white coat like a vestment, and I'd have to play the role of congregant.

Yet here I was, sweating grotesquely through my button-up shirt and my snappy slacks. It didn't seem like a good start.

When the surgeon walked in, he sat abruptly at his desk and angled the computer's monitor up, covering half his face. He asked me questions, typing my responses on his black keyboard with both forefingers. I waited for him to look up, hoping he'd meet my eyes, but he didn't.

After a half hour of his finger-pecking the keyboard (and of my wondering how someone whose job required fine motor skills had not yet learned to type), he asked, "Any questions?"

"Given all the risks," I asked him, "does it make sense to go ahead with the surgery?"

He wheeled his rolling stool around to where I sat and finally looked me in the face.

"Do you have a religious preference?"

I sat in silence for a moment. How to answer that question—"It's complicated"? And why did he want to know?

"Christian," I blurted out. It was at least a historically accurate response.

He nodded and looked as though he was scanning his mental template of responses for an appropriate choice. "Then you should seek wisdom in prayer. Ask God to guide your decision."

I understood what he was getting at: pick a god. Any god. This doctor wasn't going to give me an answer.

In the Old Testament, a man named Gideon isn't quite sure what he's supposed to do about the pesky problem of his mortal enemies. He isn't thrilled about going out to battle, but thinks that maybe he's obligated.

Gideon's at a loss, but luckily he has some animal fleece that he lays out on the ground with the intention of divining his deity's will. If the wool is soggy with dew the next day, he decides, then God himself wants Gideon to fight. The soggy fleece decides for him.

I have plenty of wool socks, and sometimes they lie out on the floor where I've dropped them and don't have the energy, will, or balance to pick them up, but they tell me nothing.

A relative who is an anesthesiologist—and a good one—drove with my husband and me to the hospital on the morning my chest was to be split open like that of a Christmas goose.

I grilled him about things I'd read when I'd scrolled down too many inadvisable pages on WebMD. Would anyone try to use contraindicated anesthetics on me? I knew it meant I could wake up on a ventilator, assuming I woke up at all.

"No one who made it past their board exams would dream of using paralytics on you," he said. "It's not something to worry about." Still, I worried.

After the paperwork and the weighing and the repeated questions as to whether I could be pregnant, the anesthesiologist arrived by my gurney and pushed a consent form into my hands. She told me to sign. The way she leaned in, jaw set hard, made her look like someone who'd played a lot of volleyball in college. I could picture her lunging forward in a dive and shouting at her fellow players to back off from what was hers.

I held the blue ballpoint pen lightly, frightened to use it just yet. I said I was sorry but that I needed—for my own panicked mind—to double check that she'd reviewed the great swath of notes from my other doctors. That she wasn't going to use any of the under-no-circumstances, totally-not-okay paralytic drugs on me. Was she?

She gave me a look somewhere between annoyance and amusement. "Of course I'm going to use the paralytics. Now you need to sign." She jostled the clipboard and its release forms at me again.

As if on some kind of practiced cue, I cried. Explosively. It was as though I'd acquired an ability to weep projectile tears.

"I do this every day," she told me.

"On patients like me?"

"A few."

"And nobody's died?"

"Not yet," she said. "But let's not put that out into the universe today."

The universe.

The *universe* was going to make medical decisions on my behalf.

She put a facemask over my nose and mouth. "It's only oxygen," she said, and in a moment I was gone.

As a teenager, when the first sparks of neurological disease started to glitter away in my body, my legs would collapse for no reason.

I was dating a church boy at the time. He wanted to be a pastor one day, as well as a doctor and a missionary. Such are the bizarre aspirations of youth. He spent his weekends watching televangelist shows. He put his hand to the TV screen when the preachers told him to, and interpreted the static crackle as a sign. He sang when he was told to sing, stood when he was told to stand. He knew he had the power of God in him, he said.

He would put his hands on me in the way that teenaged boys put their hands on girls, and he would pray.

He'd look up at me with a confused tilt of the head, wondering why it hadn't worked—why I wasn't healed.

In the neuro-ICU, it was the chaplain who frightened me the most. The man-handling doctor who wanted to enact a medieval-sounding procedure on me was hard to take, of course, but I could hear my husband standing behind me in the semi-dark of the room, saying *No*—refusing for me what he knew I would refuse for myself. They couldn't knife me or pump out my blood as long as he held his ground.

But the chaplain, when the care team sent him in, seemed to signify something worse. Shouldn't he be with a dead patient's grieving family, or with someone barely tethered to life? Then I understood.

My husband couldn't very well say *No* to a small and unassuming minister, but still, I didn't want him there. He was one more reminder that the doctors, those lesser gods robed in their scrubs and always washing their clean, clean hands of me, were passing me off to a higher power once again. An invisible one to whom it was so easy to assign a will, a plan, an out.

He asked me if I wanted to pray with him. I told him, *No.*

Not content to leave me unministered to, he tried for more small talk. He got it out of me that I taught English. He loved poetry, he told me. Did I like Wallace Stevens?

"A Rabbit," I said. It took some time to get enough breath back to add "as King of the Ghosts." Always answering these lesser gods when called upon, too afraid to tell them I didn't want any more of their attention.

The chaplain didn't know that poem, but he thanked me. Said he would read it sometime. Finally, he shuffled off to some other patient's room, and I looked for it—the poem—behind the swelling in my brain.

The difficulty to think at the end of the day,

It came in pieces, in fragments of line. My nurse walked into the room and dimmed the lights.

The whole of the wideness of night is for you,

He pushed another merciful syringe of pain killers into my IV. My skin hummed across the hospital bed, the division between my body and the white sheets blurring.

A self that touches all edges,
You become a self that fills the four corners of night.

As the heart rate monitors beeped and the IV clicked, I grew light. When I closed my eyes, I thought I could feel myself rising from where I was tethered by electrodes, lines, and tubes of every color and description.

higher and higher, black as stone—[8]

I rose, the edges of my self crackling against the darkness of the room. I rose against the doctors, small deities of these halls, and the orderlies who served them. Against their signs and wonders, against hands placed on me in prayer or in cutting. I spun into the blackness like a Catherine wheel, sparks breaking out against the night, against the silent dark, against every god who'd see his people slain.

OUR NHS
One Sick American in England's National Health Service

Notes from an Increasingly Small Island

Late on a Thursday night in June, I got out of bed and walked directly into a wall.

I staggered back, sleepy and stunned. I'd knocked myself pretty nicely in the forehead and bashed my knee well enough to form a lump that I was sure would be many shades of blue and purple in a few hours.

Why in the world had I done that? I couldn't remember why I'd gotten out of bed.

I climbed back under my comforter, still wincing and perplexed, and went back to sleep without ever recalling why I'd gotten up in the first place.

When my alarm went off a few hours later, I clicked open the BBC News website and read a headline that England, the country I'd emigrated to the year before, had voted to leave the European Union.

I felt like I'd hit the wall a second time. Why in the world had they done that?

If there's one thing that Americans are excellent at doing, it's constructing elaborate fantasies about the ways in which life is better outside the United States. Election years are particularly fruitful for idle chatter about moving to Canada, of course, but a perennial favorite for left-leaning folks like me is to recount all of the wonderful things we've heard about an enlightened and progressive Europe. If we believed our own gossip (and it seems that, often, we do), we might believe that tuition at universities the continent over is approximately five bucks per year, that people work no more than one day per week without any reduction in productivity against their American counterparts, that those inclined to have children receive 92 paid years of parental leave, and that all citizens have permanent access to petting zoos full of small and cuddly animals.

I admit it: I, too, had my leftie fantasies about what life in England would be like: I was ready to live in a country that valued tolerance. One where police don't have guns, and don't shoot unarmed black men in the streets. A country where citizens don't have guns, either, and don't slaughter one another in movie theaters, schools, or offices. A country where women's reproductive freedoms aren't the subject of endless political posturing and negotiation but are instead understood as basic rights. A country where people like me don't have to fight an uphill battle for basic access to health care despite our complex and expensive medical issues.

Like most things in life, the reality of England was a great deal different from what I'd built up in my mind. While my friends back in the United States worried about what the rest of the world would make of our hideous, humiliating, and unfortunately enduring Donald Trump interlude of national politics, the British PM installed its new Foreign Secretary, Boris Johnson. To give you a taste of his style of diplomacy, Johnson has published in his regular columns a few bawdy limericks involving the Turkish president and bestiality as well as slurs against black people that I'm not about to reproduce here. He has claimed that President Obama holds anti-British leanings because he is black, and famously called Hillary Clinton a "sadistic nurse in a mental hospital."[9] While the US installed Trump in the highest seat of power, England placed his political doppelganger in its highest diplomatic position for a period of time with no expiration date.

The dream of a society with a civilized discourse was only the first to crumble; the England in which I arrived was one in which anti-immigrant sentiment raged. It was true that gun crime was low, but knife attacks and street brawls killed people in my city seemingly daily. While local police may not have been shooting black citizens, tasering them to death wasn't out of the question. Abortion providers saw the same kinds of harassment and picketing as did their counterparts in the US, and the National Health Service, the nation's socialized system under which I was to receive my medical care during my time in the United Kingdom, was so drained by increased demands on its resources and by budgetary shortfalls that it had reached a point of crisis.

In fact, in the days and weeks leading up to the UK's nationwide referendum vote, a special election in which a simple majority of eligible voters would determine whether the UK would continue its membership in the European Union, the financial strain on the NHS became a key campaign point. NHS funding was a particularly hot topic for the group who termed themselves "Leave" (shorthand for the campaign for England to exit the EU) and for the nationalist, anti-immigrant UK Independence Party (or UKIP, a single-issue political party dedicated to extracting the UK from Europe). The pro-Brexit camp went so far as to paint a message about the NHS on a red, double-decker bus, termed the "Brexit Battle Bus," which it drove around England and used widely in publicity photos. The side of the bus read, 'We send the EU £350 million a week. Let's fund our NHS instead.' (I'm taking editorial liberties by properly punctuating and capitalizing those two sentences, by the way. The original was, shall we say, grammatically idiosyncratic.)

Voters in the UK took the bus ad seriously—the financial stability of the NHS became nearly as hotly shouted about as immigration, and was among the most prominent issues in the news media as voters took to the polls.

There was only one problem with the Brexit bus's claim: it was flatly false.

In the days immediately following the EU referendum, even the most ardent Leavers began to walk back their NHS claims. In an interview with Nigel Farage, ITV interviewer Susanna Reid pressed the then-leader of UKIP on the bus's claim:

SR: The 350 million pounds a week that we send to the EU … can you guarantee that's going to go to the NHS?
NF: No, I can't. And I would never have made that claim …
SR: Wait a moment. That was one of your adverts.
NF: Well it wasn't one of my adverts.[10]

No one, it seemed, wanted to take credit for the ad's misleading claims that a Brexit vote was essentially a vote to fund the NHS; while newspapers and pundits repeatedly demonstrated that the £350 million claim was mathematically impossible, the official website of the Leave campaign had quietly taken down much of its content. In place of its previously prominent NHS funding claims, the site now simply had a large message at the top of the screen which read, "Thank You."[11]

Thanks indeed. By autumn, the UK—helmed by the freshly-minted Prime Minister Theresa May—was preparing to enter talks with Europe to finalize its departure from the Union, and the NHS was facing a £22 billion budgetary shortfall.[12] NHS hospitals were forced to cancel much-needed hospital appointments and even operations to stay above rising budgetary waters.[13] Trends only worsened as winter set in: a December report showed that NHS operations were being routinely axed—over 400 people were denied urgent surgeries in November of 2016, a number not only the highest on record, but also double that of the past year's figures for the same period. And as the flu season approached and norovirus outbreaks shuttered entire wards across the country in the week of Christmas,[14] the occupancy rate of beds in such wards as pediatric critical care was at over 88%, a record-breaking level that forced the NHS to bus critically ill children across the country to receive care.[15] And under the country's latest funding package, rural hospitals will lose their emergency-room services, stroke and trauma care, and physician-led maternity care, forcing patients in need of such services to travel untenably long distances to receive treatment. Some areas will lose their local hospitals altogether.[16] The situation is so dire, says the Red Cross, that it constitutes a "humanitarian crisis."[17]

And as for the Brexit battle bus? Greenpeace has since acquired the vehicle. Now its advertisement reads "Time for Truth."[18]

"You Get Some Medicine However You Can"

When I arrived in the UK with two big suitcases and a lot of optimism, I was woefully uninformed about how the NHS worked. I understood the format of the system as a whole—that it was a taxpayer-funded, socialized system in which every legal resident has access to the same free, quality care—but I couldn't dredge up much information about how I would access that care. I spent more afternoons than I'd like to talk about on the project of combing the internet, looking for an *NHS for Dummies* sort of guide that would explain how on earth I would go about finding a doctor, getting my existing medications refilled, or even getting an NHS patient identification number. Even the exhaustive (and somewhat exhausting) NHS website—snappily named *NHS Choices*—wasn't much help for a neophyte like me.

I threw myself on the mercy of Sue, the international relocation consultant assigned to us by my husband's corporation. While Sue's main task was to help us find a decent apartment in London (a trickier task than it sounds: for the same price as I paid on a mortgage on a three-bedroom house in notoriously overpriced Seattle, I could, if I was lucky, get a one-bedroom mildew farm in a third-floor walkup that featured, for extra thrills, no handrails on the staircase). Even if she couldn't find us a dreamy flat, surely, as a native Brit, she'd be able to tell me where to start with the NHS.

As we sat on a bus bench for a rest after a few disappointing flat viewings, I probed her for as much first-hand information about the NHS as I could, short of asking to view her family's medical records. *How do you find a doctor? How do you get an appointment? How do you get your medications?* I felt a bit like an elderly person handing her grandkid a satellite television remote and saying, *Can you show me how to work this thing again?*

Sue laid out the basics for me: first, she said, I'd have to register with a General Practitioner—a GP. The rough equivalent of family practice doctors in the US, GPs, who serve particular geographic areas of a city, handle all the basics of care and refer patients out to consultants (what Americans call specialists) when appropriate.

That didn't sound so bad, or even very exotic. Sure, I'd be bound to whichever GP my neighborhood offered rather than free to select a doctor for myself, but I could live with that.

Sue leaned over and whispered to me, as though someone might hear her, "They're quite horrible, you know."

Maybe this wasn't so promising after all.

Sue told me the story of a friend who broke his jaw in a taxi accident just before Christmas. His GP told him to come to the office for an appointment in the new year.

I did the math—even if he'd broken his jaw on Christmas Eve, he'd still have had to wait nine full days before seeing the doctor. "What was he supposed to do all that time?" I asked.

She shrugged. "Had a miserable holiday."

I had no doubt that he did.

"Always wear your seatbelt in the black cabs," Sue said, pointing at me with her bottle of water. "That's the first thing. And when you're ill, you get some medicine however you can."

Get some medicine however you can? Images of supply runs in *The Walking Dead* came to mind. Sue was making it sound like I'd need to do a recon on the local pharmacy. Maybe I'd need to lay in some plaster of Paris just in case I needed to set my own broken limb sometime during the Christmas holiday.

A few weeks later, when I popped into a pharmacy for some odds and ends, the conversations I heard around me seemed to bear out everything Sue had said. In an aisle behind me, one woman consulted with another over how best to rid herself of a cough that, if the noise she made in the next aisle over was any indication, was either the call of a northern goose or a nasty chest infection.

"Rub some pine tar into the soles of your feet at bedtime," one woman told the other. "You'll be well by morning."

Pine tar? I peeked over the row of unguents and shampoos and the spray-can deodorants inexplicably beloved among the English. In the next aisle over, the woman was holding a jar of what looked like the worst molasses imaginable. Had these women not heard of the germ theory of disease? Was there a box of leeches on offer here, too?

But as I scanned the shelves, I began to understand why someone who appeared to be an otherwise well adjusted member of society might resort to folk medicine and pine tar after all; there weren't many products available that could be described as actual medication.

In the first aid aisle, there was no Neosporin (I'd later learn that topical antibiotics are a GP-prescribed drug in the UK) for cuts, and not even isopropyl alcohol (too dangerous: someone might drink it) or hydrogen peroxide (someone could use it to make a bomb) for cleaning up scrapes and grazes. The shelves were well stocked with salines and tea-tree oils in various preparations, but God help the person who picked up an skin infection and had to wait several weeks to see the GP for a little triple antibiotic ointment.

The cold and flu aisle wasn't looking much better. For chest infections, there was no Mucinex to exorcise those snot demons so accurately rendered in the product's US television ads. Cough medicine came only in two varieties: "tickly cough" and "chesty cough" (the active ingredient in the first being sugar, and in the second, menthol; anything stronger might be too dangerous to put into the hands of any average man on the street).

For allergies, there was no Allegra (unsafe) and no Benadryl as we in the US know it (diphenhydramine is sold only as a restricted-access sleep aid in the UK). For seasonal allergies, one could sluice one's sinuses with a foul-smelling vegetable cellulose powder blasted from a small canister, but that was about it.

For any other complaint a UK resident might have, vitamins and herbal supplements would have to do. The remaining aisles of the store held shelf upon shelf of berry extracts for toe fungus, ferns and thistles for infertility, vitamins to keep one awake or put one to sleep, and neon-colored beverages to "promote vitality." So this was what it meant to *get some medicine however you can*: find a way to achieve a placebo effect against your better judgment while you wait to see the GP.

.*. *.* .*.

KELLY DAVIO

The GP and Me (or, "You Get Some Medicine However You Can," Part 2)

In the several months it took me to settle into UK life, I'd learn that navigating the NHS isn't so different from dealing with Social Security in the US: someone gives you a number when you're born into the system, you cross your fingers and hope that your unique number isn't going to fall into the hands of people who might use it for ill, you pay your taxes along the way, and one day, when you need to use what you've paid for, you'll have the pleasure of sitting on hold on the phone with a lot of different people who will attempt to explain to you what the hell is going on.

If you're coming into the system later in life, nobody—even if they genuinely would like to help you—can say how you should go about getting a number, paying said tax, or finding the phone number to call so that you can sit on hold.

Yet after a number of false starts, phoning a call center of Glaswegians who thought I was some kind of clown for not knowing the difference between a National Insurance number and a National Health Service number, and causing a great delay and no small amount of offense by filling out a form using standard capitalization conventions rather than block capitals, I managed to get myself established in the NHS system.

At my new patient appointment at my neighborhood GP, I got my first taste of why someone might come out of a pharmacy clutching a bottle of tar rather than furnished with medication. At first, nothing seemed out of the ordinary about the appointment, other than the fact that I simply sat down in the waiting area without having to produce identification, proof of insurance, or other sheaf of documentation. She weighed me, measured my height, took down my list of current medications, and consulted Dr. Google for the British equivalents of my American drugs. We were rolling along nicely until we came to the lynchpin of my myasthenia gravis regimen: a heavy-duty immunosuppressant that, while often used to curb transplant rejection, is also useful in patients like me.

This drug—the one without which my immune system would continue to rampage against my nerves and muscles—was something she just couldn't give me. It would need routine blood monitoring, you see, to keep track of my white blood cells and my liver function.

I was perplexed; my veins were no strangers to the regular phlebotomy that accompanies immunosuppressants. Why couldn't she monitor the blood?

52

Well, you see, she couldn't possibly. And one doesn't simply. And Americans shouldn't come to the UK expecting. (That last one was quite a zinger—the suggestion that I was somehow nationally or ethnically unsuited to obtain a course of treatment routinely prescribed to other patients in the UK.) I would need to have my neurologist do all the monitoring, especially since she was in another council of London (a division roughly synonymous with a borough). Monitoring blood results should fall to the neurologist's NHS budget, not the GP's.

I'd inadvertently stumbled into a turf war, born of austerity, simply for having such a rare disease that the one clinic serving the whole of England's south happened to be in another council.

It would take dozens of phone calls, just as many emails, one tearful visit to a patient advocacy desk in the hospital's waiting lounge, a stop-gap US supply of the drug flown back to me by my husband who'd gone to America for a business trip, and four more months before I brokered a peace accord between my neurology clinic and my GP. It was a bargain that involved my travelling three hours round-trip once per week to have my blood taken, but it was a bargain that I would take.

Drug Me (or, "You Get Some Medicine However You Can," Part 3)

Anyone who's needed prescription medication in the United States knows that getting sick is downright expensive. When chronic conditions that require lifelong treatment come in to play, it can be crushingly so. One of my drugs—just one—has a list price of $805 for a 30-day supply. Another costs $213, another $267. That's not even the half of it, but it's simple enough to extrapolate additional costs from there; start tallying up a large array of specialty medications, some of which have no generic versions available, and it's not hard to see how simply staying alive can be a massive strain on any household's budget. Even for those who have good prescription insurance coverage, getting together enough cash to throw at several-thousand-dollar-strong deductibles takes about as much planning (and leaves as little room for error) as launching a satellite into orbit.

So imagine how knocked out I was to learn—once I'd finally twisted enough arms to get my medications, that is—that, under the NHS, the charge for a one-month supply of each of my prescription drugs would be just £8.40. That amount is just about $11 US. That charge applied to any medication, regardless of the type, dosage, the brand, or the manufacturer.

It was as though the NHS understood that medicine is a necessity, not a luxury item exclusively for the wealthy. Maybe they even understood that keeping people as healthy as possible keeps them out of doctors' offices and hospital emergency rooms and thereby reduces strain on the medical system as a whole. What an idea.

Imagine my further amazement when the young man working behind the desk in my neighborhood pharmacy told me that I was still overpaying; he pointed me toward the correct page on the dreaded *NHS Choices* website where, for the equivalent of about $130.00, I purchased what was essentially a season pass to medication. Any time I walked into my pharmacy, I could show them my certificate, and they'd hand me my enormous paper sack full of drugs all nestled in their delightful little blister packets (the UK is big on blister packaging, which, when you've got coordination like mine, is a real step up from childproof bottles).

Later, I'd learn that I was entitled to pay still less; a handful of medical conditions that require medication by the truckload—myasthenia included—are covered by a medical exemption to payment. What a world. I chose to stick with my prepayment certificate; I could afford it and didn't want to take unfair advantage of a payment exemption no doubt meant to help support people unable to generate an income due to disability while I was still able to work. Yet the comfort I felt in knowing that such an exemption existed was something I'd never experienced in the US.

The entire NHS medication system left me feeling generally warm and fuzzy. I didn't even mind the oddities in the arrangement that meant that each month, I'd need to phone my pharmacist so that she could send a fax to my GP so that my GP could send a fax to the pharmacy to hand over a refilled medication. I didn't even mind that it would typically take a full week for the process to go through, or that the sweet guy behind the pharmacy counter could rarely understand my thick West Coast American accent well enough to catch my surname, or that the medications always seemed to be lying in big blue plastic tubs on the floor for reasons I couldn't understand. I was getting my treatment, I could afford it, and no change in my job status or my income level could pull it out from under me.

Yet the more I learned about the NHS system, the more I realized that I was among the luckiest of sick patients, likely because my drugs were relatively cheap for the NHS to provide (even if those blood tests added up). Patients who need more experimental or costly drugs—often the very sickest patients—don't have things so easy at all.

A prime example of such unequal access to drug care stems from the recent controversy over the breast cancer drug Kadcyla. Patient advocacy groups say that the drug can give cancer patients an average of nine months more to live than standard treatment alone, and with few severe side effects. The drug is especially suited to a group of women facing breast cancer at a young age, for whom a nine-month extension of life could presumably represent an opportunity to spend precious time with their young families. But the drug comes at a price of about £90,000 (a bit under $110,000) per patient per year of treatment; the National Institute of Health and Care Excellence, or Nice (a body something akin to the Food and Drug Administration in the United States) rejected the drug for NHS use, though it is routinely used when approved by private insurance plans. Money, of course, was the key factor in the NHS's decision; the system simply didn't think the benefits of life extension outweighed the costs.[19]

Near the end of 2016, the UK's beloved AA Gill, a veteran restaurant critic for *The Sunday Times,* put a personal face on the problem of funding cancer treatment under the NHS. Gill had what he called "the full English": a particularly aggressive case of lung cancer. Gill wrote of wanting to stick with the NHS for treatment, rather than seek out private care, out of respect for the "human connection" fostered under the NHS.[20]

It's an un-American idea, this notion of human connection in the medical setting. We have, of course, the tear-jerking commercials raising money for St. Jude's Children's Hospital, not to mention those ghastly fun-runs to raise money for the highly questionable Susan G. Komen Foundation. Such heartstring-tugs go some way toward making us feel that we're in it—whatever *it* may be—together. Yet writing a check to an organization that will ceaselessly send junk mail is something quite different from the experience of truly having one's health outcomes bound up with the fortunes of others in a single, unified system on which every resident relies.

While some of us Americans are lucky enough to like our doctors, or to be treated with a little dignity when we're at our most vulnerable, our perspective on health care remains, at root, transactional. We drain our bank accounts into the void of medical billing, and we hope that, in return, we'll live. But we don't expect kindness. We certainly don't factor human relationships into our care decisions. We look at our outcomes, not our experience along the way.

But it's the very sense of dignity that I've come to understand as a particularly decent, particularly British ideal in health care. Gill himself put it this way:

It seems unlikely, uncharacteristic, so un-"us" to have settled on sickness and bed rest as the votive altar and cornerstone of national politics ... (but) The NHS represents everything we think is best about us ... what really sticks in our hard, gimpy, sclerotic hearts is looking after each other. Turning up at a bed with three carnations, a copy of *Racing Post*, a Twix and saying, "The cat misses you."[21]

Yet Gill found, at the end of his too-short life, the unhappy irony of the NHS. While the important human connection was there for him—he reports in the same *Times* column that his infusion nurse wept with him after his chemotherapy failed—the most advanced medical treatment wasn't. The UK, with its worst-in-Europe cancer survival rates, would eventually let Gill down. Nivolumab, an immunotherapy readily available to all patients like Gill in first-world medical systems, wasn't allowed under the NHS.

By the run date of Gill's final column, the very one from which the above quote derives, he was already dead.

On Strike

Cancer was on my mind when I made one of my many long trips down to King's College Hospital in South London where my neurologist wanted to see me about a suspicious-looking set of blood labs. My labs consistently turned up inconsistent results, ones we needed to better understand. "We don't want to be thinking about lymphoma," my neurologist said. Indeed, we didn't.

Outside the hospital gates, I had to squeeze my way through a picket line to get inside the facility. All along the sidewalk separating the hospital's westerly campus from Denmark Hill Road stood picketers with posterboard signs, cranked-up boomboxes, even some NHS-blue balloons bobbing in the cold air. I had arrived on the morning of an unprecedented strike of England's junior doctors.

Roughly the peers of interns and residents in the US medical system, the junior doctors of the NHS system had staged a series of industrial actions intended to force the UK government to renegotiate the new contract that it offered to its NHS workers.

The contract's terms were for a salary increase of 13.5%, a reduction of overtime pay for work on Saturday mornings and afternoons with increased overtime for Saturday nights and Sundays, as well as a pay premium for all weekend hours for doctors who work at least one Saturday each month. Other provisions included pay protections, a significant reduction in hours worked per week, and the institution of a watchdog to ensure safe working conditions in NHS facilities.[22] The British Medical Association declared the contract suitable, but junior doctors voted to reject it by a significant margin and planned a series of strikes to force the government back to the bargaining table.[23]

The public were left perplexed about just what the junior doctors aimed for. A good deal of ink has been spilled in the opinion pages as to why the junior doctors continued to strike. Many have speculated that doctors have a general concern over a growing public and governmental interest in moving the NHS to a seven-day-per-week system, rather than a weekday-only system, to help meet growing patient demand.[24] Junior doctors, it seems, weren't enthused about a seven-day system, even with protections that kept them from ever having to work more than one weekend shift in a row.

As much as my natural tendency is to support labor and hold collective bargaining as a kind of sacred action, I couldn't help but wonder silently, with a pang of probably justified shame, whether Jeremy Hunt (the much-hated NHS Secretary) wasn't on to one of his better ideas when he suggested that the UK might do better if British workers put in as many hours as Americans.[25]

I wasn't alone; a number of UK residents felt their sympathies for the doctors stretched by April's unprecedented strike action. For the first time in the NHS's history, the striking doctors refused to provide even emergency care for the sickest and most gravely injured patients. Senior staff and nurses were forced to abandon their usual duties and flock down to emergency departments where they ensured that critical cases were treated with some degree of adequacy.[26] As a result of the strike, more than 100,000 NHS patients had their operations and outpatient appointments canceled.[27] Those appointments included everything from post-operative follow-ups for open-heart surgery patients to much-needed scans for patients facing issues as serious and time-sensitive as brain tumors.[28]

I was among the lucky patients; my neurology appointment hadn't been given the ax. I and my fellow lucky ones had to squeeze, elbow, and otherwise extrude ourselves through the striking junior doctors, our eyes full of the cigarette haze they left lingering over the *we want a safe NHS* signs they held aloft.

Investigate Me

The junior doctors eventually came back to work (though similar strikes would continue on and off for the rest of the year), but those blood test results of mine never got much better. My white blood cells oscillated wildly between too high and too low, my cell volume plumped and shrank, and my red blood cell count waned eerily with every blood draw. It didn't matter whether I was well or had a cold, drank alcohol or was abstained entirely, ate my veggies or waged an all-out war on the holiday mince pies, had my blood drawn by Mary in her fashionable horn-rimmed glasses or the charming Lloyd who complimented my accent and played me Al Green records while he filled vial after vial—nothing seemed to explain any of the fluctuations that left my graphed results looking like scattered birdshot along my neurologist's chart.

I'd need to be looked at by a hematologist, my doctor said. My blood wasn't like anything she'd seen before. So off I was referred for another three-month wait for an appointment, my blood results providing ever more curious puzzles for the doctors-in-training who shadowed my neurologist and peered at my charts over her shoulder.

When my hematology appointment was about a week away, I received a large envelope in the mail. It was from the hospital, and I assumed that the contents would be forms to fill out and a medical history to notate before my visit. I made a cup of tea—that's how far my British assimilation had gotten to date—pulled out a pen, and sat down at my kitchen table to go over the documents. When I unsheathed the stack of papers inside, I was gobsmacked: these weren't routine medical questionnaires at all, but a legal warning. The hospital was cautioning me that I was under suspicion.

Not everybody in England's entitled to health care under the NHS, the documents said, and the hospital thought I might be illegally obtaining medical treatment as a foreign national. If I came down to the hospital again—as I of course planned to do for my appointment—I'd have to come prepared to prove myself or ready to pay for my treatment out-of-pocket.

My tea going cold beside me on the table, I read the documents over and over, trying to understand. How could my legitimacy to receive care be up for debate? I held a long-term UK visa that put me on the path to an Indefinite Leave to Remain status. I held a job in London. I paid my taxes—and quite a lot of them—to Her Majesty's Revenue and Customs. When I immigrated, I paid many thousands of pounds to the government in a "healthcare surcharge" to help offset the cost of adding a new person to the system. What more did the NHS want from me? And what had I done to be singled out this way?

I had, I suspected, proven myself an expensive patient.

I scanned the list of documents the hospital demanded to see from me—my visa, my passport, my proof of residency, and my banking statements constituting just a portion of the list. I started to laugh even as I cried; my US passport was across town at the American Embassy, as it was up for its once-in-a-decade renewal. My UK visa sat pasted across one of those passport pages. I might as well be a woman without a country—I couldn't prove who I was or that I had any right to be here. To make matters infinitely worse, I couldn't possibly pay out of pocket for the hematologist's appointment or for the many tests he'd no doubt run on my blood. Then again, my neurologist didn't want us "thinking about lymphoma." I didn't want to be thinking of myself as one of the dismal NHS cancer-survival statistics as I waited to be deemed worthy of care.

I called my husband and cried. I called my boss and asked if he, an immigrant himself, had ever come up against something similar. I wrote to a patient advocacy group and asked for advice. I asked a lawyer what recourse I might have.

Dozens of emails, phone calls and letters later, the NHS conceded what I already knew: I was, in fact, a legal resident. I would be allowed my 15-minute consultation with the hematologist.

Getting Around the NHS

One of the greatest features of NHS care—one that I sorely wish American physicians would adopt—is the post-appointment doctor's letter.

After specialist appointments, hospital visits, or medical testing, the physician overseeing a patient's care writes and mails out a letter to the GP, copying in other consultant physicians as well as the patient; everyone with an interest in what's going on with an individual's treatment plan is, quite literally, on the same page.

The letter system couldn't be more different from the non-system in the US, in which doctors expect patients to orchestrate care across medical specialties, hospitals, and pharmacies (not to mention insurance providers). While I can't understand the need for such a great waste of paper when email or an online system would no doubt do just as good a job at keeping doctors and patients organized and informed, I gladly accepted the inefficiency of paper over having to phone legions of unpleasant receptionists to beg for my own health records, or being made to pay for a follow-up appointment merely to get a look at my test results.

In true British style, the letters are charmingly polite. Each consultant that I saw (and I certainly did see a number of them during my time in the UK) began by thanking my GP for referring "this nice lady," and occasionally "this pleasant lady," to see them.

Shortly after the NHS investigation and its rich panoply of horrors, I received one such letter from the endocrinologist who oversaw my treatment for an early case of osteoporosis (one gift of many gifts of steroid drug therapy). It had been a routine and uneventful appointment, so I expected most of the usual business about "this pleasant lady" and some copied and pasted text about my next scheduled visit for bone testing in the new year. Instead, I found a note suggesting that I needed to be seen in the near future to address the possibility of a tumor in my neck.

My latest many vials of blood, it seemed, had manifested even further unusual signs. And while my hematologist's labs hadn't turned up anything that looked like lymphoma—to my and my neurologist's joint relief—here was a new, frightening possibility to worry about. The hospital would ring me, the doctor wrote, to schedule the appropriate scans.

It had been about six months since the same doctor had referred me for a steroid-injection class, a strange little workshop in which I'd learn to stick myself with emergency prednisone. Self-harpooning wasn't a skill I expected to need, and I wasn't too worried about missing out due to exceptionally long wait times. But a possible tumor felt more urgent. I wasn't sure I was prepared to wait so long this time.

Waiting is, however, an art under NHS treatment. The government asserts that patients who have been referred to specialist care have a right to start their treatment within four and a half months of referral. That's a fairly long wait time, especially for those who've been recently diagnosed with diseases that need quick attention and routine follow-up to bring symptoms under control. Quite a few patients don't receive treatment within anything close to that time frame, however; in 2015, the NHS conceded that nearly 40,000 patients didn't receive treatment within four and a half months, and over 13,000 patients had to wait for well over six months.[29]

In this hand of health poker, however, I'd been dealt one very useful wild card; I had a brand-new issue to worry about, not one proceeding from an existing condition. That meant I could use my private health insurance for the first time.

Private insurance in the UK is so fundamentally unlike its US counterpart that it's difficult to compare the two; in the US, insurance is our ticket to seeing the doctors we want, and to paying for all care, routine or emergency, specialist or general. We front our deductibles, cough up our co-pays, dig money from our health savings accounts, and cobble together the funds necessary to keep doctors paid and our bodies cared for.

In the UK, however, private insurance can't be used for routine health care—it can't be applied to GP visits, to ongoing care for existing conditions, or even for medications that the NHS won't cover. Patients who want private healthcare for any of the above had better come with deep pockets, because they'll be covering all of their costs on their own. Insurance for the UK patient kicks in only in cases requiring emergency medical treatment, stabilization after emergencies, some diagnostic procedures for potentially serious conditions, and some courses of chemotherapy in the case of cancer. In all situations, as soon as the insurer deems the patient ready, the company punts said patient back to the NHS for further care and follow-up. Insurance is, simply put, less a staple of care than an emergency stop-gap.

Despite the fact that British private insurance is so difficult to use, carrying such insurance is, strangely enough, a legal requirement for many foreign nationals living in the UK. All European Union citizens, for example, are required to purchase private health insurance during periods of time when they're not working, such as during maternity leave or when caring for a family member, or if they're self-employed.[30]

In my own case, my husband's employer provided us with private insurance, but so far, none of my variety of medical issues qualified for its use. Everything fell squarely under the category of maintenance. But after getting this new letter, I had, at least, a good case for trying to avail myself of that insurance card that had ridden in my wallet all year.

I phoned my insurer, spelled my name dozens of times—somehow I'm always incomprehensible on the phone, no matter what country I'm in— and haggled with a very brusque man named Carl. After much negotiation, Carl and I arrived at a scenario in which I'd be allowed a series of three diagnostic procedures. I wouldn't, however, be allowed to see a doctor— such appointments I'd have to pay for myself.

I had a few hundred pounds I could spare. I didn't know if I had six months to spare. I did the math, and I took the bargain.

When I told a friend about my upcoming appointment and the small triumph of having secured insurance coverage for my scans, he gave me an odd look. "Well, don't feel bad about using private care," he told me. "Just imagine that you're saving a bit of time for all the other people on the NHS wait list."

It seemed like an odd thing to say. Why *would* I feel bad about seeking private treatment? It wasn't like I was gobbling up a finite resource. Or maybe I was.

Bad-Tempered Health Tourists

My first consultation with my private doctor took place on a high floor of Northwest London's Royal Free Hospital, the same facility in which I saw the NHS doctor who'd identified the spooky, maybe-it's-a-tumor-looking results in my blood work.

The Royal Free is one of the finest hospitals in England—the same facility that successfully treated Pauline Cafferkey, the Scottish nurse who contracted Ebola virus during an aid trip some years ago. But you wouldn't surmise the quality of the hospital's personnel by looking at the building itself; the Royal Free looks like nothing so much as a tenement when viewed at a distance. The great, yellowed concrete edifice sits bumpily against the backdrop of the otherwise leafy neighborhood, its windows sporting many colors of faded curtains that make each ward look like an apartment with a sheet hung over the pane.

The interior of the building is, in places, a bit improved; in keeping with the British devotion to ready tea-and-sandwich availability, the ground floor has its bright cafés and magazine shops, and the glass edifice of the hospital lets in enough of the soft British daylight that the foyer feels something close to cheerful.

But take the elevator up a few floors to the NHS endocrinology ward, and the aesthetic goes straight back to tenement. It's not that the facility is squalid; in fact, it's about as clean as a facility can be with hundreds of people tromping through each day. The ward is simply old, battered, and crowded; the front desk, squashed into the hallway, doesn't allow room for a line of people, though the overworked staff can't help but let a line form. Chairs pack the waiting area so tightly that patients can't squeeze through when the nurses call for them. Ominous posters stapled to the wall read *Your Choice of Treatment,* accompanied by two photos: the first of a hand with an IV taped into a vein, and the second of a pair of hands in cuffs. *Stop the Abuse of NHS Staff,* the captions read. None of us, slumped in our chairs the waiting area, look capable of getting violent even if we harbored a strange desire to do so; there's someone waiting for dialysis, for a shot, for an exam that the hospital doesn't have on record. "It says right here," an inevitable tearful person will say, pointing at an appointment letter with a date and time, trying to convince the staff to just let them have their fifteen minutes with the doctor already. In trying not to notice the tears, we fellow patients scan the room, seeking somewhere to rest our gaze. Every item of furniture has its chipped corners, and every square inch of the floor is scuffed with the residue of decades-worth of shoe soles.

Nothing about this third-floor NHS ward prepared me for the twelfth floor, where I'd meet my private doctor. After turning a nondescript corner, I emerged into a waiting area full of upholstered, cushioned chairs, magazines on end tables, and potted fichus in the corner. The receptionists, all in sleek black outfits and full makeup, smiled while greeting patients (many of us foreign nationals) and pairing them off with translators as needed, then served trays of tea and cookies in the waiting area.

After registering my presence, I sat down, feeling acutely underdressed and under-coiffed. A woman across the room from me adjusted her clanking jewelry and muttered about the long wait. The middle-aged man beside me joined her in grumbling, though his variation on the theme of discontentment was that his elderly mother hadn't gotten enough sugars on her tea tray. "There's nothing worse," his mother said, giving a solemn nod of her head.

Nothing worse except for weeping for your dialysis appointment at the mercy of a receptionist nine floors down, I thought. Didn't we all feel just a little lucky to be here, seated in comfort and about to get medical attention we hadn't had to wait four and a half months to obtain? Meanwhile, downstairs, NHS patients crushed into the overburdened ward. What had any of us done to deserve better, or to earn a little cookie tray as we waited? We had nothing but luck cut with cash.

This was what AA Gill later called "a plush waiting room with entitled and bad-tempered health tourists,"[31] the very thing he wanted to avoid by sticking with the NHS in all of its gritty, populist glory. The NHS isn't just about waiting, it's an exercise in patience. It's not just getting what you need; it's a reminder that everyone deserves medical care and equal treatment. Opt out of that egalitarian, all-in-this-together environment, and what we're left with is peevish entitlement.

Now I understood what my friend was getting at—what guilt I'd have to stave off if I wanted to get private care. When I entered the consultation room to meet my doctor, I understood it even more: my endocrinologist was a doctor I recognized from my visits to the NHS ward. He wasn't someone who practiced exclusively on this posh floor, but was instead an NHS doctor making time to see patients apart from his NHS schedule.

When he sent me off for my tests, it was the NHS facility that the radiologist used as she performed an ultrasound on my neck. It was the NHS phlebotomist who drew my blood. It was down on the NHS endocrinology floor that I picked up the additional testing supplies that I was to take home with me. Here I was, a private patient, using the premises of the socialized system. I tried to remember my friend's advice: maybe I'd actually let someone on the NHS have my spot on the waitlist. I couldn't shake the feeling that perhaps I'd just used my money to jump to the front of the line.

A Pronoun Says So Much

When this pleasant lady received her letter from the fancy private practice, the results of the scans and tests were deemed inconclusive. The private doctor was bouncing me back to the NHS, my letter said, for additional studies. I was no further along in my diagnostic odyssey now than when I'd begun; I was merely £400 poorer and feeling a little inconclusive myself about whether I'd made a good choice.

Quite a few UK physicians would say an unequivocal *no*. Doctor John Dean, an Exeter cardiologist, recently wrote a scathing view of private doctors' practices in the *British Medical Journal*. Dean says that he himself can no longer countenance practicing medicine privately; in his experience, private consultation amounted to little more than doctors finding expensive procedures and treatments for which to bill patients (a practice that we American patients aren't unfamiliar with). "I was involved in a business where the conduct of some was so venal," Dean said, "it bordered on criminal—the greedy preying on the needy." When it came to private medicine, he concluded, "for most 'ordinary' private patients … the main advantage is simply to jump the NHS queue."[32]

Despite the fact that patients are likely to overspend on private care and that queue-jumping disadvantages fellow patients, reliance on private continues to grow; patients spent £13 billion on private medicine in 2016 alone, a figure that represents a 76% increase over such spending in 2010. It's not hard to see why patients are forced into the choice—"efficiency" cuts to the NHS have reduced the system's capacity by over five million patients per year, the number of professionals willing to practice on the frontlines of the NHS as GPs and nurses is shrinking, and waitlists for care are at an eight-year high.[33]

If those indicators don't point to a bad enough problem for the NHS, there's another crisis looming for the NHS; the system employs many doctors who live and work in the UK as foreign nationals. These doctors, many of whom have given decades of service to the system, may not be allowed to remain in the country after the Brexit ordeal has finally concluded. That's a concern that could easily drive doctors to leave the country early, on their own terms, rather than wait for the government to give them the boot. And the said looming boot isn't mere speculation or baseless fear that's leading doctors and patients alike to panic over the doctors' right to remain in the country; the Prime Minister herself is leading the rhetorical charge against foreign workers in the NHS. When asked by the BBC whether NHS doctors from foreign countries will be allowed to stay in their roles, PM Theresa May replied,

> There will be staff here from overseas in that interim period—until the further number of British doctors are able to be trained and come on board in terms of being able to work in our hospitals. We will ensure the numbers are there. But I think it's right that we say we want to see more British doctors in our health service.[34]

Our health service. That pronoun says so much. I used to think, when I first came to England, that the British tendency to refer to the NHS as our health service was a charming one—one that valued the patience and goodwill that keep the system running, that reflected the all-in-this-together sprit of the health service.

It may be that, as AA Gill says, the NHS still represents the best of us, but it remains to be seen who that us will be. Will it be those who can pay to opt out of a system buckled by high demand? Those who live in urban centers rather than underserved rural areas? Those who were born in England and not subject to investigations—or even revisions—of their legal rights?

It's an unfortunate likelihood that, with such limited resources, heavy demand, and a double-down on austerity measures from the government, the UK could see its health service dismantled in favor of a privatized system—one that looks a lot like the very broken one in the US. All of the right pressures are in place to squeeze out social care in favor of private-payer care; we all know how quickly ours can become merely another term for mine.

III. ON DISPLAY

IF WE LEARNED ANYTHING
FROM DAVID BOWIE

On the morning the world learned that David Bowie had died of cancer, nearly every person on my Underground train had open a copy of the local paper, its front leaf showing Bowie in his younger days, all sparkling glory. The carriage was Ziggy after Ziggy, the headline announcing his death so startling that we seemed to assimilate it only through repetition. *Blackstar* streamed in the cafés and pubs, and flowers piled in a memorial on a Brixton sidewalk.

Tributes came sweeping across social media, too. For a few days, it seemed that the entire world was grieving, taking comfort in being part of a chorus of voices that offered condolences, gave gratitude, and registered shock. But as always seems to happen, after the initial sting of the news, the editorializing began. The headlines claimed that this newly passed icon of ours wasn't so important after all, or that his finances or views on copyright were somehow lacking and in urgent need of discussion.

Strangest of all, at least to me, was an opining tweet that claimed, "If we learned anything from David Bowie," it was "that cancer can be private."

I had to stop and read again. Surely I was missing something. We weren't about to forget the bottomless well of creativity, the power of self invention and reinvention, or the decades of art-making, were we? We weren't about to wash over Bowie's contributions by saying that the great lesson of his existence was that he chose not to talk publicly about his diagnosis ... were we?

In the following days, as the first sting of the news faded, I'd see many more such statements creeping up across media of all kinds: more bizarre praise for Bowie's closed-mouth policy about his cancer. I wondered what were other cancer patients supposed to make of this public rallying in support of non-disclosure.

I myself haven't experienced cancer, and I hope I can live out the rest of my life saying so. I hope all the people I love and—in a Pollyanna-ish way, given statistical realities—all those reading this can do likewise. But even as someone on the outside, I suspect that, if there is one thing cancer patients don't need, it's a pack of strangers judging the merits of their highly individual choices on what to say or not say about their diagnoses.

No, I don't know what it's like to deal with cancer. But I know how it feels to live with a disease that kills some while sparing others, has no cure, and comes with some highly toxic treatments that, together with the disease itself, affect every aspect of life. And I know what it's like to face the twin pressures that affect all sick people: to be inspirational, or to be quiet.

If you are going to disclose your illness, our culture tells us, you had better do it in such a way as to make other people feel gratitude for their own good health, to take advantage of their robust bodies, to dredge up whatever peppy feeling they get from that horrendous "I Hope You Dance" hit of the 90s. It typically involves a great many 5K runs with graphic t-shirts, and words like "battle" and "courage" used liberally. The brute facts of your existence should make others feel lucky not to be *you*.

The inspiration path is an exhausting one for the person trying to travel it; it's less about a positive attitude than it is about performance art. The energy it takes to look put together rather than disheveled, to keep from crying when you receive the news that a promising treatment isn't working, to speak like a broken record of your hope for a cure when what keeps you awake at night is the fear that you might not wake up—that all takes more energy than many of us have.

It's really no surprise that some—especially someone like Bowie who was already so exposed the public's prying interest—choose to say nothing at all. If you don't have the stomach to deal with others' demand about what your experience should look like, do you have any choice but the privacy of silence?

Of course, you could choose to speak plainly about the circumstances of sick life in the same way that others discuss frustrations with work, troubled marriages, or money problems. But here's where disclosure gets sticky: talking about illness turns out not to be like talking about those issues at all. Talk about a bad boss or a bad partner and that's *venting*. It operates on the assumption that these are experiences that most people hold in common; it acts as a mirror that nearly everyone can see themselves reflected in.

But when you talk about a bad body, that's *complaining*. That's asking others to relate to something they don't want any part of. That's to become a grim image in a mirror held up to mortality. Keeping quiet, then, can be just as much about others' comfort as those fun-runs are.

And something I don't imagine that all those people praising Bowie's silence-as-heroism realize is this: long illness comes with its own terrible sort of privacy, and it's neither freely chosen nor ennobling.

In my case, I've developed a ferocious brand of interiority born of the hours, weeks, even months I've spent largely alone. As my muscles grew weaker and I lost the ability to use them normally, I had to cut back further and further on the number of hours I spent teaching until eventually that number hit zero. Soon I couldn't breathe or speak well enough to chat with friends on the phone, much less meet for a social gathering. As my world grew smaller and my close friends less numerous, I aimed my loneliness at books—both the reading and writing of them. But when my eyes couldn't track words well enough to read a page, and when my muscles were too wobbly to allow me to write for more than a few moments at a time, I retreated even further into the solitude of my own mind.

That privacy was perhaps the greatest loneliness of my life.

I was grateful to shed that solitude for a couple of years when the trend of my health moved in a positive direction. Thanks to some frightening yet effective treatments, I regained enough strength to work again, to write, to spend time with others without rationing strength to pay for every word or breath. I almost forgot what it felt like to be that alone. But when that familiar feeling of bonelessness in my legs returned, and when even my eyelids began to drag down again as if under extra force of gravity, I felt that my allotted time in the wider world was slipping into the past. And I could feel my life folding in on itself, like a slip of creased paper, sliding slowly back into envelope after envelope after envelope.

When I think about David Bowie and the cancer diagnosis that so many praised for "privacy," I say a kind of retroactive prayer that he didn't experience the loneliness, the quiet and long and inexorable drawing into the self. I hope the end of his life wasn't private at all.

KYLIE JENNER
AND HER GOLDEN WHEELS

I saw it first in a train station: the poster of a woman who looked like a contemporary Marilyn Monroe ascending a staircase. Her platinum hair was sleeker than anybody's I'd ever seen in windblown London, and her black dress hugged her the way every woman imagines a dress one day will but never does. What interested me the most about the image, though, was the fact that, as she turned her head over her shoulder and threw up a saucy eyebrow at the camera, she balanced on a pair of forearm crutches—standard-issue aluminum with cuffs and handgrips. I don't often see depictions of women using mobility aids looking powerful and fashionable, so I stopped in the middle of the mob shoving toward the train and looked a little longer.

Flanking the woman were two beefy bodyguards in what I took to be designer suits. The men braced the woman, holding her up on either side, as though without their help she'd tumble down the stairs. At the bottom of the shot were the model's feet, trussed up in a pair of strappy platform heels.

The debilitating condition that put her on crutches, the viewer is meant to understand, was the height of her designer shoes.

Talk about a letdown. What I'd taken for a badass image of a woman unapologetically occupying space with mobility aids was something else entirely. It was just one more advertisement suggesting that women manipulate themselves in some way or another in order to look pretty. Which is to say, another advertisement, period.

I adjusted my pair of sneakers and started slowly up the stairs in the Underground station, grabbing onto the handrail so that I wouldn't take an actual tumble on my actually less-than-mobile legs. I didn't have any bodyguards in Armani suits to hold me up, after all.

After seeing that ad, it probably shouldn't have surprised me to see Kylie Jenner—she of, well, inexplicable fame—striking her own disappointing pose a few weeks later when she appeared on the cover of *Interview* magazine.

It's an odd enough choice for a stylist to give such a young woman a hair-and-makeup combo that make her look like she's about to sing "Blue Velvet" in a David Lynch film, but never mind that—the most bizarre feature of the photo was that the able-bodied girl, shiny in her latex corset, sat perched in a golden wheelchair. What would possess a healthy, abled person to have her picture taken in a wheelchair—one from which she's free to hop up at any moment—I couldn't say, but if you believe scores of supportive fans and their internet chatter, the image was meant to symbolize her *limitations*.

I don't claim to know what limitations Ms. Jenner has experienced in her life, but I feel confident that they have nothing to do with wheelchairs. Or with canes or walkers or hearing aids or any of the other devices people use to get on with their lives. These aids are tools of freedom in the world, after all, not markers of restriction.

So what was this image of Kylie-in-the-gilded-wheelchair really about? The same thing the image of the woman with her precipitous shoes was about, I suppose: the idea that's its somehow edgy or provocative to see a beautiful woman with the visible signs of disability. The idea is that beauty and disability are opposites, and that it's artistic to juxtapose them for effect.

In short, it's about the notion that the atypical body is typically sexless and unappealing, and that to look at such a body otherwise is pleasurable only if it's lurid. It's an idea rarely spoken but widely accepted, and here it is, printed on glossy paper and packaged to sell.

Yet we don't have to buy it. Most considerate people recognize that popular culture has a body image problem, and that we do women and girls serious harm when we celebrate certain body shapes while devaluing others. Unfortunately, that realization has given us a new obsession: looking "healthy" is our new substitute for looking thin. For those of us for whom looking well or able is just as unattainable as, say, heaving our way into a pair of size-zero jeans, that supposedly positive message isn't positive at all.

Perhaps it's time to recognize that we do women just as bad a disservice when we put too high a value on outward appearances of health. All of us deserve to move confidently in the world just as we are—not cast in the shadow of someone else's gold-painted wheelchair.

GIRLS ON OXYGEN

Oxygen is delicious. I'm not talking about fresh air—I'm talking about oxygen straight from the tank, pumped right into the nostrils through plastic tubing. You've got to be willing to overlook the new-shower-curtain smell, but as soon as the gas starts flowing, the thoughts come into focus, the vision clears, and as long as that nosepiece stays wedged up the nostrils, it's less of a struggle to be in the body.

I didn't realize that oxygen tanks were also increasingly fashionable until I'd spent some serious time with one after major surgery. In the weeks after leaving the hospital, I had more time than energy, so I did what any self-respecting convalescent would do and binge-consumed media. It was after some long hours spent with A&E's series *Bates Motel* and the "must-read" book of last year, *The Fault in Our Stars,* that I learned that every sick girl in pop culture needed, like me, her very own oxygen tank.

Bates Motel follows the life and exploits of a young Norman Bates in contemporary Oregon. The series focuses squarely on Norman—who will grow up to keep his mother's desiccated corpse in his living space in *Psycho*— painting him as a kind and well-meaning (if troubled) teenager. But more interesting to me than the sympathetic, maybe-he's-misunderstood portrait of Norman is the perplexing treatment the show gives his sidekick, Emma. She's got good looks, smarts, a dry sense of humor, and style that suggests a personal shopper combing vintage stores on her behalf. But, God help her, Emma's also got a thing for young Norman.

Emma's problem, though, is that she's also got cystic fibrosis (which the show's producers signify by popping a nosepiece on Emma and giving her a charmingly tiny oxygen tank to wheel behind her). Actress Olivia Cooke gives a dry little cough every few episodes to remind us of Emma's diagnosis, but otherwise, Cooke's Emma is a vision of health. We even see her execute some pretty impressive sprints through the Oregon forest, tank in tow, the absurdity of which would've made me laugh if I'd had enough lung capacity to manage it.

It doesn't matter what kind of wit, personality, or forest-navigation skills Emma has—her illness is a deal-breaker for Norman, who is, naturally, focused on the popular, able-bodied, yet emotionally unavailable Bradley. Silly sick girls, *Bates Motel* tells us, even corpse-hoarding Norman Bates isn't going to love you.

The Emma storyline isn't disappointing because it's unexpected; in fact, the characterization's as trite as any on television. What's disappointing is that the *Bates Motel* writers had a real opportunity with Emma. She plays such a major role in the narrative that she could very well have been her own person instead of a cardboard-cutout sick girl—the writers could have allowed her some personal ambitions, say, or the opportunity to develop meaningful relationships with other characters. Instead, they're content to let her moon around the motel, hounding for Norman's affections, ready to aid Norman in whatever low-grade quest he has in each week's episode.

But the writers do, from time to time, take Emma's oxygen away from her. We catch her in moments when the tubing is off her nose, and we are supposed, I presume, to catch our collective breaths about how pretty she'd be *if only,* and to mumble *what a shame.* But this quick-change trick is as goofy in *Bates Motel* as it is in David Lynch's *Twin Peaks* when Maddy, Laura Palmer's cousin, takes of her windshield-sized eyeglasses and suddenly, in soft light and with an orchestral swell behind her, she's a knockout.

The easy-on, easy-off special effect of the oxygen tank troubles me not just because it's such a lazy production trick; it's also because it suggests that being sick in a publicly visible way is somehow a shame, and that we sick girls would be better off and easier to accept—even love—if nobody had to see us dragging around our accoutrements.

On the other side of the oxygen-tank-as-prop phenomenon in pop culture are strangers who are a little too comfortable with sick-girl paraphernalia, and who assume that girls like us must make great educational resources. John Green's *The Fault in Our Stars* (I'm a sucker for an sale-priced ebook) features another girl equipped with an oxygen tank: Hazel, a teenaged girl living with cancer, who makes herself inexplicably available for other people's passing interests.

Hazel is at least the heroine of her own story, not a sidekick like Emma in *Bates Motel,* but she too has to earn her keep around healthy people; when accosted by a curious child in the local mall, Hazel removes her nosepiece and lets the child wear it, explaining that the oxygen helps her scarred lungs to function a bit better. In what's supposed to be a charming scene, the little girl announces that she, too, feels much better now. After the teaching moment concludes, Hazel gives the plastic nosepiece a wipe on her shirt and pops the fitting back into her own nostrils as the child shuffles off.

I had to put the book down after reading that scene. Frankly, I wanted to take a shower, or at least to make very liberal use of hand sanitizer. Hazel is, like me, taking high doses of steroids. While they have many wonderful therapeutic benefits, steroids suppress the immune system, significantly reducing the body's ability to combat infection. For the person taking a high-dose steroid, a germ as innocuous as that of the common cold can precipitate a rapid spiral into pneumonia. A flu virus is even more serious business. A disease like whooping cough, which is making quite the comeback thanks to vaccination skeptics who put others at risk for the sake of their ill-informed opinions, would almost inevitably mean lights out for Hazel.

But Green seems to think it's fine for Hazel to willingly place her personal medical device in someone else's germy, mucousy nostrils for the sake of satisfying a toddler's curiosity. For Green, the satisfaction Hazel experiences at the interaction appears to be worth the very real risk to her health. If she's going to die anyway, the book suggests, her job in the meantime must be to teach healthy people some friendly life lessons.

It's not fair, of course, to expect that the every fictional representation of sick women be accurate reflections of the many and varied aspects of our lives. Maybe I should just be happy to see, for once, some characters who resemble me. But I think it's fair to want to see those characters treated not as sad cases or as life-enriching educational resources but as *people*—human beings made up of the same stuff as everyone else, occupying the same space as everyone else, breathing the same air, even if it comes through a plastic tube and a nosepiece.

THANKS A LOT, *MIAMI INK*

In my mid-twenties, I sat for my first and only tattoo. It's a sizable piece on my left shoulder: a wax-sealed envelope nestled in a bed of primroses. In my mind, it was a reminder that, regardless of the bad news of life—rejections, failures, royal screw-ups—good news would come for me, too. There would be acceptances, success, and plans that came off well. It was a simple little affirmation, one I still appreciate from my past self, and it was a beautiful design.

After having wanted the tattoo for some time and having researched what seemed to be every artist in the greater Seattle area, I felt proud of my new ink the way I suppose a project manager feels proud of coordinating a team's efforts. All I'd done was pick the right person and sit without squirming for the three hours it took him to get the ink into my skin; the artist did all the hard work, from the drawing and stenciling to the placement and execution, but I still loved showing off his efforts. Strangers would stop to comment on the beautiful way he'd used color, or ask who'd done the tattoo. I was always happy to direct people to his shop and evangelize his talents.

As I got older, paler, and more likely to nestle myself away in the traditional Seattle all-season hoodie than to wear a spaghetti-strapped top, those conversations stopped. At times I even forgot my tattoo was there. Unless I caught sight of it in the mirror as I got dressed, I had little occasion to think about my reminder, my emblem.

Yet when I got sick, I learned about one of the lesser known side-effects of illness: having to get naked (or mostly naked) in front of strange people on a startlingly frequent basis. In fact, it's a rare treat to go into any medical office and not be told "it ties in the back" as someone chucks a sad old gown in my direction.

And so for the second time in my life, my tattoo's become a topic of conversation. Only now nobody's telling me that they like the line work or asking for the name of my artist. Now people want to hear a good story.

I suppose "What's your tattoo mean?" seems like a good ice-breaker—

at least it's more original than asking how the week's been just to break the silence. "It means I have a tattoo" seems like a perfectly good response to me, as does "What does your receding hairline mean?" But then, I want to be a good patient.

I suppose I can't be too hard on these nurses, assistants, and physical therapists with their passing curiosities. Americans have been trained to assume that every tattoo has a story—a story we're invited, simply by having seen a glimpse of someone's body art, to hear. We lived, after all, through the pop cultural growing pain that was *Miami Ink*, a show that taught us that every tattoo should be accompanied by a harrowing story.

Miami Ink's producers seemed to prefer narratives that involved unlikely survival—the kind of thing fit for a *Reader's Digest* "Drama in Real Life" feature. Tragedy was acceptable, too, especially if the word "family" could be repeated with high frequency. To my eye, the images people chose to have inked on their skin and the narratives they told about those images bore little relationship to one another. At best, they employed an entirely private system of symbolism ("this skull with bloody daggers coming through the mouth represents the special bond I had with my grandmother!").

I admit to having watched enough episodes of the show to understand what people are after when they ask about my tattoo. I try to give them a good story. I work in "strength," sometimes "courage," all while wondering when the forced, clinically necessary intimacy of having to undress for strangers—strangers who will prod upon the body with gloved hands and any number of implements—became so confused with actual intimacy.

A person's literal nakedness shouldn't imply emotional openness. It doesn't give a person the freedom to ask anything, so why do I always offer up a story on demand? Why not redirect the phlebotomist's line of conversation to what he's having for lunch, or tell the nurse practitioner, in manner of Jennifer Aniston in *Office Space,* that "I don't really like talking about my flair"?

It's because, unfortunately, I need them. In this balance of power, they're on the heavy end of the scale. They're still the ones with the white coats. They hold the needles. They write the orders. As long as they make me strip bare before the scalpel, the reflex hammer, and the electrode, I'll tell them anything they want to know.

SICK GIRLS WILL OUTLIVE EVERYONE IN THE COMING ZOMBIE APOCALYPSE

Aside from our mutual interest in keeping me alive, my neurologist of many years and I do not have much in common. He's the sort of guy who takes vacations to go shoot at wildlife on the tundra. I, on the other hand, still get creeped out by eating runny egg yolks. I have a sneaking suspicion he's of a libertarian bent while I was pant-suited up for a Hillary Clinton presidency. He wears a fishing vest much of the time for reasons I couldn't begin to guess at. He finds the fact that I still sometimes insist on tottering around in high-heeled shoes equally perplexing.

But there is one thing we hold dearly in common, and that's our joint enthusiasm for all things related to the zombie apocalypse. It's not unusual for us to go over a previous week's episode of *The Walking Dead* while he prods at me with spiky instruments, and I typically arrive early at my appointments so we can chat over which new apocalyptic paperbacks he's reading. If he weren't so busy with the likes of his patients, the man could, I believe, edit *The Year's Best Zombie Fiction*.

He recently told me about a new title that featured a character with, of all things, myasthenia gravis—the same rare neuromuscular disease that he's treating me for. We had a laugh over the similarities between the way I walk on one of my worse days and the way a TV zombie waddles, though I maintain that I am still much cuter with my shuffle. Our conversation made me think, though, about the fact that it's incredibly rare to see or read about a character with any kind of debilitating condition in the never-ending stream of pop-culture zombie scenarios.

On the surface, a lack of us special cases on the post-apocalyptic scene makes sense—anybody tough enough to survive a pandemic-level virus must be specimen of good health, or so I suppose the thinking goes.

I'm not so sure, however. If anybody's got the skill set to avoid a zombie-making virus, it's those of us who, year after year, navigate flu season with suppressed immune systems. If anybody's going to be able to out-maneuver a walking corpse, it's those of us who daily make our way through public spaces that are as rife with potential danger as a forest brimming with the undead.

In fact, I think that sick girls will outlive everyone in the coming zombie apocalypse. You'll never meet better tactical thinkers; we know which hours of the day we can go to the grocery store without running into a teeming horde of toddlers who'll try to kick our canes out from under us (a weekend salvo on Trader Joe's is frankly excellent supply-run preparation in this regard). We know with eerie precision how many steps it'll take to get to any marker in a room, and we can plot the best courses to conserve our energy. We are excellent at picking out which person on any crowded bus or train is most likely to whip around while wearing a giant backpack, smacking us in our faces. We are never taken by surprise.

Sick girls also know how to keep our food from killing us. We grill our lettuce, boil our bananas. We know that the unassuming grapefruit is really Satan's softball, ready to interact spookily with any medication imaginable. We hydrate as though it were our paid profession, and our handbags are veritable pharmacies.

I can further guarantee that sick girls' sanitizing game exceeds that of anybody on *The Walking Dead*. I know I'm not the only person who shudders when the otherwise delectable Glenn relieves a zombie of its head with his machete, then wipes a brain-covered forearm across an abrasion on his brow. Glenn, the sick girls of the world are here for you. We will minister to you with our Wet Ones and our Purell. We carry antibacterial bandages with us at all times, and we will let you have as many as you want. We are even fairly certain we could cajole the overripe Darrel into a soapy bath. At the very least, we have travel-sized Lysol spritzes that we can use on him.

Something tells me that, all of the above notwithstanding, we're not likely to see more of our sickly selves in pop cultural images of the world's end. It's a lot more enlivening to watch a powerhouse like Maggie Greene putting a piece of rebar through a walker's eye socket than it is to watch girls like us waddle a well planned and clear path through the forest. That's okay. We'll let you have your Maggie for now. But when the zombie apocalypse arrives, stick with us.

EMPIRE GOT IT WRONG

In the coming months, Fox is expected to renew for yet another season its wildly popular show, *Empire*. The drama centers on Lucious Lyon, fictional music mogul, record executive, and bad guy of Shakespearean proportions who spent the show's first season believing he was dying of ALS. Yet in the last few moments of the finale, a smiling neurologist tells Lucious he actually has myasthenia gravis, and that it's "highly treatable." Shortly after, a home nurse gives Lucious an unidentified shot and tells him that, within a short period of taking these injections, he'll be symptom-free.

Hours after the *Empire* finale, bloggers were writing their hot takes on Lucious and his revised diagnosis. *Slate* summed up Lucious's new reality by saying he has "something non-life threatening called myasthenia gravis."[35]

To me, a myasthenia gravis patient, the idea that I have "something non-life threatening"—and that there's a magically curative shot nobody bothered to tell me or the medical establishment about—comes as news.

Someone else who might be surprised to hear from *Empire* that myasthenia gravis isn't life-threatening is the actual artist, songwriter, and producer Stephen Ellis Garrett, who was diagnosed with MG seven years ago.

You might not recognize Garret's name, but you've almost certainly heard his music. Garrett, who wrote, produced, and performed as Static Major, worked heavily with Timbaland (who, if you've been watching the credits closely, you'll recognize as the executive music producer for *Empire*), collaborating on '90s touchstones like Ginuwine's "Pony"—which has found new life in the *Magic Mike* movies—and on Timbaland's remix of the Destiny's Child hit "Say My Name."

Static backed Jay-Z on "Change the Game" and wrote "Can I Take U Home" with Jamie Foxx. He's the songwriter behind Aaliyah's success—he wrote her hits like "Try Again," "We Need a Resolution," and her final single, "Rock the Boat." He's featured on Lil Wayne's crossover hit

"Lollipop." And that lo-fi vocal on Drake's "Look What You've Done"? That's Static's voice, sampled from an old home video.

But we can't ask Static what he thinks of the way *Empire* handled MG. In February of 2008, Static was admitted to Baptist Hospital East in Louisville, Kentucky, for treatment, and he didn't leave the hospital alive. He was only 33 years old.

You could be forgiven for thinking that MG is no big deal if you relied on *Empire* for information. The most difficulty the disease seems to give Lucious is a wobbly hand while he tries to shave one morning and a quick bout of hazy vision while he plays piano. His symptoms last no longer than a few seconds at a time, and they don't, frankly, seem any more serious than a hangnail.

Reality couldn't be more different.

Here's what actually happens to a person with MG: communication between nerves and muscles breaks down. That breakdown causes muscles— important ones—to stop working properly. If Lucious were a real patient, one of his eyes would likely droop or close completely. He might have trouble speaking above a whisper, and singing would almost certainly be out of the question. He'd probably be frustrated by spending so much time at his bar, Leviticus, because he might not be able to swallow well enough to get a single cocktail down. He'd probably have difficulty walking normally, much less striding through his office like a god.

He'd definitely have to take a whole cavalcade of pharmaceuticals just to get through the day, and some of his pills would work for only three, maybe four hours at a time. Some of his drugs would likely be chemotherapy standbys, and the side effects exactly what one expects from chemo. If he were very lucky, Lucious could potentially go into remission, but odds aren't in his favor.

That's the easy stuff, the day-to-day living. The worst of MG—the part that patients like me and Static have had to experience—is something *Empire* doesn't even broach: MG also affects the muscles needed for breathing. When muscles grow too weak to allow a patient to breathe adequately on his own, he's said to be in a *myasthenic crisis*, and is usually placed on a ventilator to keep him alive while he undergoes additional treatments.

One such treatment is plasmapheresis, a procedure in which a high-volume catheter—a device that looks like it came out of an *Alien Versus Predator* movie—is implanted in a patient's neck. Or, hopefully it is.

82

Sometimes the catheter goes astray, puncturing a lung or giving a patient a hematoma. Over a period of several days, all his blood is pumped out through this catheter and effectively scrubbed clean of the antibodies causing his symptoms. And he'll be awake and alert for the whole, painful process.

It was during plasmapheresis treatment that Static died of respiratory failure.

In the video Drake sampled for "Look What You've Done," Static stands before the camera, the lens close in. He looks almost shy despite the fact that he's a powerful man, a kingmaker among artists who perform his songs. He says, "Music is," and pauses. "It's like breathing."[36]

Static didn't want to undergo plasmapheresis. His wife Avonti told Phillip M. Bailey of *Leo Weekly* in 2009 that her husband was crying during the procedure. "I'm not feeling them fucking with my arteries," she remembers him saying.[37]

I understand that sentiment. When I found myself in the ICU during my first myasthenic crisis, the neurologist insisted I have the catheter implanted in my neck immediately. All I could say—whisper, really—was "I can't."

Later, when I could speak again, I tried explaining myself to the attending doctor. "I couldn't handle it psychologically," I said. "Plasmapheresis—it's barbaric."

He looked at me for a long moment and nodded. "*Most* of the treatments we have to do are barbaric."

Watching Lil Wayne's "Lollipop" video, it's hard to imagine that Static—flanked by beautiful women in the back of a massive limo, singing poolside at a Vegas villa and wearing a designer suit, upstaging Lil Wayne with his effortless cool—would be dead just weeks after the video shoot wrapped. But Avonti, in the same *Leo Weekly* interview, said that she noticed her husband's speech slurring when they talked on the phone, and that he reported being unable to open his right eye. She said that his breathing sounded so labored it seemed he was choking, and that he was so weak he came off a Louisville flight from Atlanta in a wheelchair.

That's how quickly MG can move—how insidious it is. By the time the "Lollipop" video debuted, Static had been dead for over two weeks.

That's what *Empire* wants you to believe is no big deal. That's what Lucious's doctor is talking about when she says myasthenia gravis is "highly treatable."

In the US, there are just 70,000 of us with MG. That may sound like a fairly large number, but compare that with the nearly three million breast cancer patients in the US and you begin to get a sense of just how rare a disease we're talking about. That rarity is an obvious plus for *Empire's* writers; it's easy to play fast and loose with the details of a disease that few people have ever even heard of. The show's creatives feel abundantly free to whip up a fictitious shot that Lucious can take to be magically cured. Who's going to call foul, after all?

The problem, though, is that now we patients have to live with the misinformation that *Empire's* spreading; it's difficult enough to navigate daily life with a body that, when it's at its worst, is barely functional. We don't need the added wrinkle of having our friends, acquaintances, and coworkers brush us off as malingering with "that non-life-threatening thing that Lucious Lyon was cured of."

Nobody's saying *Empire* has a duty to realism. This is a show, after all, that featured a rival record company hacking the Empire office's elevators through the magic of the internet. Its characters write fully realized, perfectly harmonized duets on the spot. Everyone is beautiful. Everyone is talented beyond believing. We watch *Empire* for the drama, the music, and the fantasy, not for clinical reality.

And I'm not asking for gratuitous portrayals of suffering—I don't need to see Lucious drop dozens of pounds because he can't swallow food, or see him totter when he has to stand unaided. I don't need to watch him walk with a cane or stop being able to carry a tune because his diaphragm is too weak. I don't need to see his body broken in all the ways mine's been broken just to feel seen.

What I am asking for is that *Empire's* writers demonstrate a little bit of responsibility. I'm asking that they not wave away myasthenia with fictional and impossible treatments that belittle lives like Static's, or like mine. I'm asking that what we have to live with—from life-threatening symptoms to lack of safe and fully effective treatments—be handled with a little compassion. It might be too much to hope that Timbaland use his position as executive producer to honor his late colleague Static's music, but I hope for as much anyway. If we real patients can't get a dose of Lucious Lyon's cure-all shot, at least give us that much.

ON REPRESENTATION

Toward the end of August, I traveled to Edinburgh to catch the end of the annual Fringe Festival, a month-long celebration of theater, dance, comedy, music, spoken word, and street performance that takes over nearly every corner of the city. Some of the shows are gems, while others are duds; the programming is voluminous, uneven, chaotic, and on the whole, wonderful.

I was particularly eager to catch some theater; for me, there's nothing equal to the transporting power of a play, and there were some promising offerings that weekend. The first production I settled in for was an adaptation of Henrik Ibsen's 1894 *Little Eyolf*. I have a soft spot for Ibsen and his heavy-handed moralizing, and was eager to see what this adaptation might do with one of his final works.

The play turned out to be a student effort that treated us to some unusual decisions: a giggle-inducing translation ("What a joy it is to be a road worker!"), a young woman who took her top off at regular intervals for no apparent reason, a Sufjan Stevens track running through some needlessly complex set changes—you get the idea. But it was the Fringe, after all. Student work happens. I was onboard for whatever these folks wanted to do for the next hour or so.

At least, I thought I was. My feelings changed when the title character, Eyolf himself, came onstage.

Eyolf, for those unfamiliar with the play, is a nine-year-old boy with the long-term goal of becoming a soldier, and with the more immediate passions of learning to swim and watching the local rat-catcher at her work. He uses a crutch because he has one paralyzed leg. The original text of the play describes Eyolf as having beautiful, intelligent eyes.

What came clattering onto the stage was anything but the character that Ibsen had written. What emerged from behind the curtain was a large puppet.

Someone in the theater company had constructed a grotesque, child-sized doll using jointed wooden dowels for limbs and what appeared to be a paper mâché bowl for a head. The person playing Eyolf's mother manipulated the puppet from behind, and spoke all of his lines as though through the featureless, stark-white head-bowl.

I felt my stomach coil in on itself. Was this some kind of gross joke? I glanced around the rest of the audience, my face no doubt contorted in the universal expression for "Are you seeing this?" I didn't find that look reflected on any of the other theatergoers' faces. The character of a disabled person was being played by an inanimate object, spoken for by the character's parent, and we were all, apparently, going to pretend that it was okay.

I hadn't expected this show to provide the most nuanced portrayal of disability I'd ever seen. But I had expected the play to—at a very low minimum—feature *a human being*.

Like a lot of disabled people, I've gotten used to the fact that we rarely get any representation onscreen or on stage. Even when roles do exist for disabled characters in films, shows, or stage productions, those roles are almost always filled by able-bodied actors—ones who are lauded for their "sensitive" or "brave" portrayals of what disabled actors who are denied those roles experience daily. Yet nobody, even those who rightly call into question casting choices that put white actors in minority roles (see the conversation generated by Emma Stone's playing Allison Ng in *Aloha* for one recent example), seems to care about whether actually disabled people get to play themselves.

For a long time, I couldn't understand why that was the case. If it's creepy and weird for Stone to play Ng, surely it's just as creepy and weird that Stone is slated to play the Rosemary Kennedy—disabled by a heinous and forcible botched lobotomy—in the upcoming film *Letters from Rosemary*.

Yet over time, as I saw critics heap praise on able-bodied actors playing disabled roles, I began to understand. It was the way that reviewers couldn't help but gush about these actors that showed me what a lot of people really think of disabled folks: when Eddie Redmayne starred as Stephen Hawking in the film *The Theory of Everything*, *The Guardian* said that "to look on as his face and body distort is to feel, yourself, discomforted, even queasy."[38] Or when Daniel Radcliffe played Billy in the alarmingly-titled play *The Cripple of Irishmaan*, a *Chicago Tribune* reporter Chris Jones said that Radcliffe "delivers a Billy with one heck of a limp, a body-twisting contortion that, when in motion, is quite the theatrical thing to behold."[39]

These reviews would be laughable if the truth lurking behind them weren't so disappointing: the sight of disabled bodies is distressing enough to viewers that they'd prefer not to see the real thing. Worse still, the presence of able-bodied actors allows viewers a pass in voicing how disgusted they are with our "distortions" and "contortions." No one (I hope) would say they feel queasy at the sight of model and actor RJ Mitte—one of the rare, actually disabled actors on television—playing Walter White's teenaged son Flynn in *Breaking Bad*. Surely no one would write that his body is theatrical to behold in its motion. But (I fear) they're thinking it.

With such a mentality at work in the world, I've had to accept the idea that I'll never see much screen or stage representation of people like me. Allowing disabled actors to be cast as themselves on a regular basis is a social development I don't think I'll see in my lifetime. Yet I have to draw a line at puppetry; to suggest that a blank-faced doll with rattling dowels is good enough? That's something nobody should accept.

IT'S JUST NERVES

I've never seen *The Little Mermaid*. Ditto *The Wizard of Oz*. File next to *Ghostbusters*. I've never read the *Chronicles of Narnia* or *Alice in Wonderland*. The Smurfs, Care Bears, and My Little Pony were names we didn't dare speak in my childhood home, even if commercials for their Hasbro-produced toys and breakfast cereals punctuated the few television programs I was allowed to see.

My sister and I had to settle for Bible videos—ones that reenacted some of the more G-rated scenes from the Old Testament—that our mother checked out from the church library. The repetitive nature of God-saves-the-day plotlines was tedious to me even as a six-year-old, but there was no point in complaining; I wasn't going to get access to the good stuff. In our family's off-brand version of Christianity, any pop cultural product that carried even a whiff of magic or fantasy was strictly forbidden. At best, reruns of *Betwitched* glorified sorcery. At worst, books like *A Wrinkle in Time* could irrevocably warp the moral consciousness. It wasn't because such stories and the characters in them might be too scary for a young kid (after all, we saw more frightening displays on the Trinity Broadcast Network all the time as televangelists shouted about Armageddon). Instead, it was because these shows and books were downright dangerous.

God-fearing is what my family might have called itself, but what really worried us was the devil. He was always lurking, always rapping lightly at the door and waiting to be let in. Anything dark, anything not "Christ-centered," as the church put it, could crack that door open, letting Satan get one foul, hairy toe over the threshold.

Even in my irreligious early twenties, I hadn't screened so much as *The Nightmare Before Christmas*. I assumed that I'd be ill-equipped to sit through anything remotely spooky. After all, I had no conditioning against dripping monsters lunging from swamps or ax-wielding murderers stalking towns after sundown. A part of me, though, wanted to see what was so frightening that it could leave someone—a person with a tenuous grasp on theology and an eagerness to believe, of course, but *someone*—thinking that a movie could create a bona fide portal to hell. I wanted to see if what I'd been sheltered from all those years was really so terrifying once it came shuffling across the screen.

As with most things in life, reality couldn't match the scope of what I'd built up in my heart. Maybe it's down to my ravaged adrenal glands, largely dormant after years of steroid therapy, but I turned out to be pretty hard to frighten. I watched film after film, but the weak sparks of what adrenaline my body could muster when baddies jumped out from behind doors or out of wrecked cars were cheap scares, and no different from what I'd get from a stranger's sneeze on the quiet car of a train. Even when I gave up on the subgenre of movie that I like to call "stuff jumping out from behind other stuff" (a genre including hits like *Paranormal Activity*), I still didn't find much that rattled me. *The Silence of the Lambs* was gross, and *Event Horizon* sticky-looking, but they weren't frightening. Nothing about the scenarios or plots seemed credible to me; I couldn't fear something so obviously fake.

It was when I finally sat down to the granddaddy of scary movies—*The Exorcist*—that I finally got the scare I was after. It wasn't because of the head-spinning and crab-walking trappings of the possession story. That was all fantasy—still that slick unreality that couldn't shake me. What frightened me was that, when I peeked behind all the set dressing and gore, I recognized myself in the film.

The Monster Arrives

The setting of *The Exorcist* had nothing to do with me, of course. I spent my childhood in a tract house on the dusty edge of Fresno, not in a sprawling mansion in Georgetown like Regan, the 12-year-old girl who's the subject of the movie. I dreamed of one day owning a pair of jeans that my sister hadn't burned through first, not of convincing my mother to buy me a horse. I'd never even seen a Ouija board in my youth, much less used one to conjure a spirit like "Captain Howdy," the demon who later possesses Regan. The distance between my life and hers elided, though, when I saw her face, slack and exhausted from sleeplessness.

I knew that face from the mirror; while Regan couldn't rest because the monster that wanted to inhabit her body shook and tossed her bed all night, by the time I was Regan's age, a monster had already moved in with me. It came in the shape of pain: a hot, restless pain in my legs and arms that wouldn't subside no matter how I twisted or shifted on my twin bed.

90

Decades later, I'd understand that pain to be the result of injuring my weak muscles over and over as I pushed, unmedicated, through daily activity. At the time, I knew it only as a nightly visitation, an ill-willed, consuming presence that chewed away at my limbs.

I recognized, too, the look on Regan's face as she told her mother what was happening—that wide-eyed expression, asking for help she couldn't give herself. I'm sure I'd worn it, too, the first time that I tried to explain the beast that came to me each night, that was getting so bad that it made me cry, made me beg God for help, that made me scream into the soundless void of my pillow.

While Regan's mother believed her daughter and rushed her to the doctor for a battery of tests, my own took her characteristic hard line, issuing prohibitions against complaining and assurances that "growing pains" were just a part of childhood. Even though Regan's plotline and mine diverged here—her story led to the doctor's office and mine to years of holding my tongue—we ended in the same place. We were fractal limbs that still branched from the same, gnarled trunk: both Regan and I were easy to dismiss.

A Case of Nerves

Regan's doctors poked, scanned, imaged, and otherwise assayed her using every method then known to medicine, which is to say that they subjected her to a variety of barbaric studies that doctors wouldn't dream of using now. She was subject to everything from a pneumoencephalogram (a gruesome procedure that involves draining a patient's cerebrospinal fluid from around the brain and replacing that fluid with air or gas bubbles) to an arterial puncture. As is so often true in life, these diagnostic procedures failed to produce any useful results. The doctors decided that Regan's trouble was simply "a case of nerves."

We'd be surprised to hear a doctor use the term "nerves" today, but up to the era of Regan's and my childhoods, such vague umbrellas ruled medical and popular opinion; for a time, anything from headaches to back pain were thought of as manifestations of neurotic tendencies.[40] Though biological explanations for physical problems eventually replaced nonspecific categories like "nerves," it wasn't until 1980 that clinical practice abandoned the use of the term "neurosis" for good.[41]

Terminology may have changed for the better, but it's not necessarily the case that doctors or the public think about illness much differently than they did in Regan's or my youth. When tests fail to turn up clear results, the presumption isn't that the tests themselves are flawed or limited, but that there's nothing physical to find in the first place. It's a line of thinking that I recognize all too well in its updated, contemporary clothing: *you're probably stressed. Have you tried deep breathing? How about yoga? You should try mindfulness.* It's an assumption that I encountered even recently when a well-meaning family practice doctor suggested taking me off life-saving medication in favor of an anti-anxiety pill (though I'd never been diagnosed with an anxiety disorder in the first place), as though she believed that a disease of the nervous system was really just "a case of nerves."

While Regan had the benefit of early medical intervention (a luxury that I would have sold my soul for as a child) and I had "tough love," a "bad attitude" and a mouth full of teeth chipped and broken from grinding my jaw in pain, our plotlines converged here, too: being disbelieved made us both big bundles of nerves, ripe for the devil's picking.

Making Room For the Devil

The gaps in what's known about the human body have always been fertile ground for superstition. When diagnostic processes don't reveal anything treatable (as in Regan's case), or when patients are denied medical assessment in the first place (like I was), it's not uncommon for pseudo-scientific beliefs to reach their sticky roots into a patient's fears. Those roots anchor everything from blog-fueled claims that fresh juice is a legitimate alternative to chemotherapy to late-night infomercials touting vitamins or Pilates as prophylactics against and cures for diseases of all descriptions. For girls like Regan or like me, whose family histories predispose us not just to illness but also to religion, those roots tap down to an older, more sinister place: the crucifix, the censer, and the splash of holy water.

It's not hard to see how it happens, this grasping for a spiritual cause for a physical problem; the influence of an unseen moral force has always been a favorite explanation for what science has yet to describe. Even if we'd like to think that our collective human behavior has improved along with our advances in the sciences, some people will always make room for the devil. Those who saw Halley's Comet in 1066 wrote of the downfall of nations in the wake of its passing, and in 1996, the Heaven's Gate cult committed mass suicide in order to be supernaturally absorbed into a spaceship that they believed flew in the wake of the Hale-Bopp comet. Ancient peoples attributed earthquakes to the thrashing of a massive, subterranean catfish or the twitching of a vast turtle, and in 2010, Pat Robertson claimed that the earthquake that struck Haiti was divine retribution for the practice of voodoo. And while we now understand that exorcism, throughout its ugly history, was primarily used as a weapon against people with physical and mental health problems, exorcism remains a regular practice in the Catholic church today.

Doctor Richard Gallager, professor of clinical psychiatry at New York Medical College, made the extraordinary claim in *The Washington Post* that the United States alone has roughly 50 Church-recognized exorcists, some of whom report being called upon for their services around 20 times per week[42] to perform exorcisms not unlike the one performed on Regan. In 2004, the Orthodox Church, another branch of the Christian faith, found itself at the center of an international media storm when a 23-year-old nun in rural Romania was killed during an exorcism. The young woman, widely known to have schizophrenia, was crucified to death.[43]

The Charismatic church, too, that freewheeling offshoot of Protestantism in which I was raised and which is known for demonstrations like "speaking in tongues" or "slaying in the spirit," sees its share of exorcisms (though Charismatics tend to prefer terms like "deliverance" and "spiritual warfare"). Because the basis of Charismatic belief is that the faithful are led not by a church hierarchy but by the spirit of God himself, the faith structure is a decentralized one, with individual practices and even principles of doctrine varying wildly among congregations; there's no oversight to any church practices, even ones as sensitive as, say, driving out Satan himself.

In my teenage years, when my pain had worsened to the point at which I imagined that my skeleton was trying to pry itself loose from muscle and tendon every night after sundown, I found myself in a particularly devil-focused Charismatic group. That church typically relied on parishioners who were said to have "the gift of discernment," a Christianized version of what secular spiritualists might term "sensitivity," to spot demonic possession. These gifted ones were, in my experience, almost always older men, though sometimes the younger men got involved, too, apprenticing themselves in the detection of the devil. But men they were, and they could spot a demonic possession wherever they looked, especially when they looked at girls.

Even more common than possession was something that the discerning called "oppression," a lower-grade demonic affliction that, while stopping short of allowing an inhuman spirit to fully control a human body, caused a person to commit all sorts of grievous sins and engage in questionable behaviors that she wouldn't have been inclined toward otherwise. Everything from teenaged drinking or compulsive gambling to buying secular records or overeating during the holidays could be the results of oppression. Those simply weren't Christian things to do. If a Christian person did commit any of those spiritual crimes, the line went, then another actor must have been at work. It was a simplistic notion, of course, and one that manhandled the doctrine of free will. Yet the appeal was clear; if we weren't in harmony with the church's teachings, we ourselves weren't to blame. All we had to do was to get rid of the demon. If we succeeded, we'd be free. We'd be at peace.

And so we looked to the discerning to tell us about our demons so that we could engage in the spiritual warfare—the exorcism rites—that would drive them out. Anybody, regardless of age or clerical status, could perform such a rite. Some of the more cavalier thinkers—even by Charismatic standards—thought that a person could exorcise himself by reciting highly specific prayers found in the backs of books on topics like "spiritual bondage."

In our congregation, it was always toward the end of the worship session that parishioners would flow to the front of the room and ask for intervention. Those old, doughy-handed men placed their palms on foreheads to drive out devils and send them back to hell. But as anybody who's watched enough horror films knows, in order to drive a demon out, first you have to know its name.

Some of those names were from the hit parade of spirits associated with deadly sins: the demon lust, the demon wrath, the demon envy. These few seemed to attend church with us regularly. But there were other visitors, too: the demon cancer. The demon multiple sclerosis. The demon Parkinson's. The demon depression.

You see, much of the Charismatic world doesn't merely blur the line between illness and spiritual depravity, mistaking the former for the latter. Instead, deliverance ministers hold that physical illness is a direct consequence of spiritual oppression. If God is good, surely he wants us to be healthy and happy. If we're not healthy and happy, then once again, an external and willful actor must be the cause. They believe that the devil quite literally makes us sick.

And so those men in our church drove him out—or said that they did—

Satan and his legion of companions. They commanded, too, that the sick be healed, so the sick claimed that they were. To do otherwise would be to deny God's power—to blaspheme. People went without their medications, skipped therapy, tossed away assistive devices that they needed for daily living, and believed.

At least, they pretended to.

Yet some of us wouldn't. Some still took their pills. Some stayed ill and visibly so. What did those men make of those of us who persisted in living in our fallible bodies after they'd put their hands on us and demanded that we be healed? We must have looked to the deliverance ministers just as green-faced, just as decayed, just as venomous as Regan did to the two priests who turned up at her bedroom door in *The Exorcist*.

That's what my family hid from behind a pile of Bible videos and prohibitions for so many years. It wasn't the devil at all—it was the truth. *The Exorcist* isn't a fantasy, but a reality that too many girls have lived: when sickness comes to stay, parents see bad behavior, doctors see nerves, and ministers see evil; no one sees little girls any longer. They see only the monsters turning our bodies into spoilage and waste. We girls don't merely break inside ourselves, but we break apart for an audience of men who come to watch, to scream at us to be healed, to be different from what we are. In the dark, after the credits roll and the film reel flaps to its end, the monster chews and chews.

IV. THE WIDE WORLD

A WOMAN ALONE

It was a small table, barely big enough for me, my glass, and the sheaf of papers I had spread out before me, but that's how I like my space: cozy, personal, not inviting to strangers. The total opposite of the long, communal tables in the middle of the pub where families sat—their kids in wellies and their dogs crusted with mud after an off-leash excursion on the Heath—enjoying their lunch before presumably going home to be hosed off as a group. I came early for this table. I know that London pubs fill up early on Saturday afternoons, and I wanted a nice corner to work in beside a long and light-filled window.

I was bent over one of my author's manuscripts-in-progress, pen in hand, when a woman with a toddler in her arms approached me, asking, "Do you mind?"

At first I thought she intended to sit down with me, stationing herself and her happily gurgling daughter at the tiny, one-person table with me. I must have looked perplexed by the question, because there was nowhere for them to sit.

Then I understood: she didn't want to share. She could have done that at any of the longer tables in the room, all with open seating for more people. She wanted *my* table, and she wanted me out of it.

I shook my head, smiled in what I hoped was a moderately polite way, and turned again to my work.

"Well, are you waiting for someone?" she asked, setting down the wriggling girl who slapped a sticky palm on my papers.

"No," I said.

She took the notion in, as though it were hard to imagine that a woman on her own wouldn't be waiting for someone.

"Well, are you just *relaxing* here?"

Frustrated now, I dropped my fake smile. "I'm working."

She gave me a sour expression as she rolled the idea over, then finally walked off.

I watched her install herself and her child in one of the communal areas. She didn't ask anyone else to move for her: only me. Only the woman alone.

Most of what I know about street harassment (or what I suppose we should just call "harassment") comes only from hearing other women's stories. I listen with sympathy and horror when they tell me about being catcalled or leered at or touched by strange men in public, but I can count on one hand the number of times I've been subjected to such behavior. I've often felt that I have a strange kind of privilege associated with having an irregular body: with my eyelid that droops and mouth that sags when my facial muscles get tired, with my puffy steroid cheeks, my always-bruised skin, and the waddling gait I often have even when I don't use my cane, it's mercifully rare that I'm subjected to unwanted sexualized attention. So far I've taken it as one of the only benefits of looking somewhat *off* that I haven't had to deal with that kind of nonsense when I venture out into the wide world.

Yet as I held my ground—or my pub seating—against the woman who wanted to know what business I had taking up space, I wondered whether harassment was a broader thing than I'd imagined. Perhaps it had less to do with the male gaze than with keeping women in line, reminding them of their place. Even when it was other women doing the reminding.

That's not something I'm exempt from, no matter how much I wish I could be.

When I'd gotten through as much editing work as I was likely to finish that evening, I decided to skip the Underground and walk home to my apartment a mile or so away. It wasn't raining, and I needed a little exercise (easy downhill strolls being my favorite thing to call "exercise").

As I came to the confluence of a residential road with the high street, I saw a sparkly Land Rover backing, illegally, into the intersection. It was dark already, and I wasn't sure the driver could see me, so I chose to wait on the curb until he and his SUV had passed by.

Instead of driving on, the driver hit the brakes, rolled down his window, and shouted something at me that I couldn't make out.

"Sorry?" I said (having learned that, in England, *sorry* can be used as a synonym for *huh?*).

"I said I have a license to drive on this road!" he shouted again.

"Okay?" I said, genuinely confused about what the problem was. "I'm just waiting for you."

"Don't use that body language with me." He was red in the face, screaming.

"What body language?" This was getting bizarre.

"That gesture with your arms!"

I had my hands in my coat pockets. Apparently, that constituted a *gesture*.

My hands, however, did not remain in my pockets. As he railed at me further, I availed myself of both middle fingers, as well as of some of the more colorful parts of my vocabulary.

Finally he drove ahead into oncoming traffic and left me to cross the street in peace.

I fumed for the rest of my walk, appalled that I couldn't sit at a table in a pub or even stand quietly on a sidewalk without having my right to take up space challenged. I arrived back at my apartment, shut the door behind me with a clunk, and stood in the dark feeling bitterly homesick.

I wasn't homesick for my life in America, for once, but homesick for a place where women are allowed to walk alone at night. To put our hands in our pockets if we feel like it. To sit at tables. I was homesick for a world that never existed.

In college, I knew a woman who used dry-erase markers to scrawl scriptural verses about "biblical womanhood" on her dormitory mirror. It was the usual business about virtue being better than rubies, covering oneself in tapestry (that sounded overly warm to me, but what did I know?), and raising up children. The point of the exercise, she explained, was to remind her not to judge herself by her looks, but by her inner being. A nice enough project, if irritating to her roommates who were trying to get their eyeliner on straight in the shared mirror.

At times I think I'd like to adapt her practice and write on the interior of my front door, in indelible Sharpie, *I am allowed in public.*

The trouble is that *I* already know I'm allowed. It's the rest of the neighborhood I'm not so sure about.

MINDFULNESS IS FOR HEALTHY PEOPLE

I was waiting on a train platform in south London after a round of tests at the hospital. It seemed like half of the city was waiting there with me, including a woman reading a giant, dog-eared paperback titled *MINDFULNESS*.

When the train barreled into the station and its doors shushed open, the woman wedged herself to the front of the line of waiting commuters, and shoved onto the train without waiting to let those leaving filter out of the car first. She elbowed fellow passengers out of the way and scuttled into one of the seats reserved for pregnant people and the elderly, all while keeping her eyes glued to the text of *MINDFULNESS*.

I'm tempted to say I couldn't believe it, but I could only believe it too well. Just a few days prior I walked passed a group of adults deep in conversation about "mindfulness" who were apparently unaware that the small child walking with them was staggering out into oncoming traffic. Mindfulness, if the way it's deployed by my neighbors is to be believed, is the practice of being so fascinated with your own wellbeing that other people cease to be a consideration.

I know, I know. The half-meditation, half-behavior adjustment technique that is "mindfulness"—when it's practiced by people who don't make commuting a full-contact sport or allow their kids to shamble out in front of delivery vehicles—is supposed to make us better, calmer, happier, more contented people, and what few studies exist on the practice seem pretty appealing. When I found myself in the stress trifecta of a chaotic workweek, a health crisis *du jour*, and an impending visit from my overseas in-laws, I was tempted enough to give it a brief, slightly ill-willed try. Or, rather, a retry.

You see, I've never liked meditating. Early on in my diagnosis and treatment for myasthenia gravis, I took up various medical practitioners' recommendations that I give meditation a go to reduce the stress that comes along with so much change and uncertainty. I sat dutifully on my little cushion, set a timer, closed my eyes, and hated every moment of it.

I had all of the common complaints: meditating was boring, I couldn't focus, and that boredom and lack of focus frustrated me. But there was something else: the obsession with "the breath." I was supposed to *feel* the breath, *follow* the breath, *notice* the breath—I didn't want to do any of those things. My ability to breathe had deteriorated along with my muscle strength, and paying additional attention to the sensation of my weakening in-and-out of air was a reminder that, in my neurologist's words, "That's how myasthenia patients die." In the end, I gave up meditating in favor of taking a good nap now and then.

So when I downloaded a goofy-looking mindfulness app to my phone to take another crack at the whole business of meditation, it felt less like an innocuous idea than a potentially unpleasant one. Yet when life involves so many medical tests with so much stressful poking and prodding and frightening results, there was something nice in the idea of achieving more calm in the face of the scary and difficult.

I clicked the app open and listened to the little beach soundscape, synthetic gulls crying over a manufactured ocean. I obediently closed my eyes, sat in the prescribed position, and followed along with a guided meditation in which a chipper narrator encouraged me to "scan" my body.

This wasn't a promising start. Any kind of "scan" of my body is something I try to avoid. As the narrator encouraged me to "notice" the body from the head downward, I had the opportunity to feel, in higher-than-desirable definition, my neck slumping under my skull's weight, my stomach chugging along with the first of five sets of medication for the day, my arm aching from too many needle-sticks in one week, my knee twisted from losing my balance on a set of stairs.

Next the narrator told me to observe the sensations of the body *without judgment*, experiencing the body without any emotional response to what I was feeling.

That didn't seem like the kind of thing I was willing to do. If "feeling the breath" and "scanning the body" were unappealing, then this non-judgment business was a deal-breaker. Sure, a bit of dust tickling the end of a nose or the sensation of a lumpy cushion under one's butt are experiences we can observe without feeling one way or another about them. But what happens when the body you bring to this exercise experiences objectively bad sensations—sensations like pain?

I shut down the app and didn't open it again. If this was what mindfulness was all about, then it wasn't for me. It was for healthy people.

For some time, I'd be unsettled by this idea that it's somehow helpful and wise not to judge what happens in the body, even when what's happening involves suffering. Surely I was missing something. I read as much as I could, looking for some suitable explanation for this idea that so many others assent to but that I couldn't sign on for.

Finally, I found a statement approximating a defense in a text by mindfulness mega-star John Kabat-Zinn:

> We speak of awareness ... as perhaps naturally 'uncoupling' the sensory dimension of the experience of pain from the emotional and cognitive dimensions of pain. In the process, the intensity of the sensations themselves can subside. In any event, they may come to be seen as less onerous, less debilitating.[44]

Ah, there it was. Another iteration of the tired—and dangerous—idea that we can think our way out of what hurts and bootstrap ourselves out of what debilitates.

We didn't need mindfulness meditation to give us this notion. Culturally we are already nothing short of a mess when it comes to dealing with people who suffer: we equate a need for pain management with drug abuse and push legislation to make necessary treatments harder for patients to obtain. We tell people to throw out their medication in favor of exercise, as though clinical depression or multiple sclerosis could be sorted out with a good squat-thrust or two. We tell others that losing weight or drinking foul-smelling juices will cure cancer or halt Parkinson's, all medical evidence to the contrary. We assume that pain and human suffering are for the weak, the slothful, the lazy. In short, we do little but judge, blame, and scold people when they are at their most vulnerable. And now we have Kabat-Zinn and the mindfulness movement to tell us that debilitating conditions can be "less debilitating" if we would just quit having emotions about them.

Maybe I'm an outlier; there may well be plenty of sick folks who take comfort in mindfulness. But I believe that it's fundamentally dangerous to treat human suffering as value-neutral, and I refuse to take part in a practice that promotes thinking, breathing, and scanning one's way out of illness or disability.

Perhaps what we need is a little *less* mindfulness—less eager willingness to "uncouple" the mind from the body—and a little more empathy for other human beings. What would happen if we invested less time in contemplating our own internal states and more time in creating an inclusive, compassionate culture? Or if, instead of suspending judgment about suffering itself, we tried instead to suspend judgment about people who suffer? Of course, there's no smartphone app for that, and no easy-to-market lunchtime seminar or coffee table book. But something tells me that, even without the slick packaging, it's worth a shot anyway.

THE STATE WE'RE IN

Perhaps the only positive thing that can be said about the 2016 US Presidential election is that it's over. This past campaign season was dreadful in a way that's not so different from dropping a cube of compacted trash on the kitchen floor: an impressive amount of rot and filth came clattering out at us, and while we'll be cleaning up the mess for a while, it's hard not to stand back, slack-jawed, and survey the slimy mess. There was the bitter primary season that divided the left into calling one another "Hillbots" and "Bernie Bros," the degrading spectacle of the Clinton v. Trump debates, and, of course, the stunning outcome of the election in the small hours of November 9. We scratched our collective heads over the FBI's late-game email stunt and tried to sort out why the right couldn't bring itself to care about Trump's hot-mic admissions of sexual assault. We wrote our names on dozens of petitions, we marched, we sought Hillary Clinton in the woods for selfies as though she were the mythical Sasquatch herself. And, predictably, we talked about moving abroad.

The run-up to every election has its share of people grumbling that "If *he* wins, I'm moving to Europe." It's usually nothing more than idle talk—an escapist fantasy that allows us to feel just a little more in control of our lives in the face of political currents that we can't change. Yet in the months after the election, I heard more and more people describing the actual steps they're taking in preparation for moving abroad: selling homes, cashing out pensions, getting passports renewed, brushing up on high school language courses.

I understand, to a point, the emotional appeal of getting the heck out. There's a particular flavor of hopelessness that we taste only when we realize that the progress that we've worked for in our communities and the causes that we've invested in over our lifetimes can be scuttled so quickly. The work to change our country for the better begins to feel as futile as it does endless, and we allow ourselves to fantasize about disappearing into a more enlightened society that will allow us to quit fighting so hard all the time—a place where somebody else has already cleaned up the social and political messes.

It would be unfair to discount the fact that there are people at heightened risk: those who have had their headscarves torn off, who have been grabbed—or worse—by men emboldened to sexual violence, who've had to comfort their children who hear chants of "build the wall" in their schools, who have no recourse as the Klan marches down their city streets, who find their homes and playgrounds spray-painted with swastikas, whose marriages are threatened with dissolution, and whose access to health care is under threat. For people in fear for their basic safety, the moving-abroad fantasy isn't so much an issue of escapism but a hope for survival.

I admit that, when I moved to Europe when my husband's job was relocated, I was eager to leave the US behind. The ugly rumbles that would culminate in the 2016 election outcome had begun even then, and I fantasized about being elsewhere: somewhere more civil, more accepting, more thoughtful, more welcoming. Somewhere, if I'm honest, I could pretend that the problems of my home country were someone else's to carry.

Brexit, and the economic downturn that came with it, brought me back to the US far sooner than I'd planned, and I brought with me an understanding that my fellow liberals may not want to hear: Europe looks a lot like home.

I arrived in the London long before then-Prime Minister David Cameron announced a public referendum on the UK's membership in the EU. The biggest hubbub in the UK's political sphere was the recent rise of Jeremy Corbyn, a Bernie Sanders analogue, to the head of Labour (the country's opposition party). Yet when Cameron announced the simple-majority vote that would determine the UK's future, the relative calm that had—I thought—prevailed began to turn into something else entirely. The country's dialogue became centered on the choice between Leave and Remain. And jockeying to position himself at the vanguard of Leave was a man named Nigel Farage.

My fellow Americans—who could have easily assumed that "Brexit" was a fried breakfast dish for all the attention paid to the referendum by the US news media in the months ahead of the vote—may know Farage as Fox News's newly-minted political analyst. Or they may have learned of Farage first when he, in the week that Trump was elected, celebrated the fact that the UK would no longer be working with "that Obama creature, loathsome individual who couldn't stand our country." As if that racially charged *creature* remark wasn't enough, in the same interview, Farage made light of sexual assault claims against Trump by joking that he hoped the new president could keep his hands off UK Prime Minister Theresa May, and suggested that May might need him as a chaperone: "Don't touch her for goodness sake ... If it comes to it, I could be there as the responsible adult couldn't I? Make sure everything (is) okay."[45]

Or they may have heard of him first during the surreal spectacle that was the "Brexit Flotilla," a slow-moving nautical skirmish on the Thames River involving Farage and a group of fisherman demonstrating for Leave in a small fleet of boats. Those boats were headed off in a surprise maneuver by a yacht owned by pro-Remain Irish singer Bob Geldof (yes, he of the Boomtown Rats and "I Don't Like Mondays") who taunted Farage with some graphic hand gestures and colorful remarks delivered over a bullhorn. A few hours and some lively business with water cannons later, and the whole display was over. We Londoners were left wondering whether the stunt that had just unfolded in front of us hadn't made D.C. politics look tame for a brief moment.

Long before, however, Nigel Farage was the head of the UK Independence Party, or UKIP. Far from standing as one of the more influential parties in the UK, the far-right UKIP doesn't even hold a seat in the House of Commons. And Farage, much maligned by establishment politicians, was considered something of a political laughingstock; Farage was the butt of every joke I heard on late-night comedy television, and perhaps it was precisely because he was so easy to joke about that he was also easy to discount. He seemed like nothing more than a brash, often offensive oddball who was so far from the locus of power that we could safely giggle at him. No one, it seemed, thought he had any likelihood of mobilizing large numbers of citizens behind him (something that may sound a bit like a person we Americans are dealing with today).

Yet Farage's UKIP attuned its message to economic concerns of the struggling working class—the party's symbol is a large purple pound sign against a gold background, if that gives you an indication of its platform— and tapping into fears about immigration. (These two tactics may also seem familiar to Americans.)

UKIP's official position is that it is not a racist party but a nationalist one. *Nationalism* is a queasy enough term for a lot of us, but Farage has also made quite a few remarks that seem directly in opposition to UKIP's claims of racial tolerance. Here's what Farage had to say in the wake of the terror attacks in Paris in November of 2015: "I think we've reached a point where we have to admit to ourselves, in Britain and France and much of the rest of Europe, that mass immigration and multicultural division has for now been a failure."[46] Farage didn't limit himself to broad comments on a multicultural Europe. He also had some close-to-home specifics to offer: "Any normal and fair-minded person would have a perfect right to be concerned if a group of Romanian people suddenly moved in next door."[47]

Yet Farage's lowest moment in stirring up anti-immigrant sentiment in support of the Leave campaign came when he unveiled his signature Brexit advertisement: a massive poster that featured an image of Syrian refugees walking down a rural road in Europe. The caption at the bottom of the poster read, in bold red letters, "BREAKING POINT." And below, "The EU has failed us all." Leavers loaded the posters on large mobile billboards and drove them around London,[48] to the great dismay of many of us living in the city. The intent of the ads—though they stopped just short of calling the refugees themselves dangerous—was abundantly clear to many of my fellow London residents, some of whom even reported them to the police as hate speech intended to drum up racial tension.[49]

Many supporting the Leave campaign continued to deny that anti-immigrant sentiment had anything to do with their Brexit push; this was about jobs, the economy, and a system that had disenfranchised the working class. But no one could ignore the racist tensions seething in the country when, on June 16, Jo Cox—a human rights advocate, Labour Member of Parliament, and an outspoken Remain supporter—was assassinated by Thomas Mair.

Mair, who called himself "a political activist" and gave his name as "death to traitors" as he was being arrested,[50] shot and stabbed the mother of two to death in the street outside her constituency surgery (a series of one-to-one meetings with area residents). Multiple witnesses to the assassination describe hearing Mair—whose internet records show an affinity for Nazi, Klan, apartheid, and other white-supremacist reading material—shouting the political slogan "Britain First" as he shot Cox once in the chest and twice in the head with his .22 Weihrauch, and stabbed her fifteen times in the heart and lungs.[51]

On June 23, the day of the referendum vote, the walkways outside Parliament were still covered by a vast, makeshift memorial with flowers and hand-lettered signs exhorting us to "Love Like Jo." And they were still there the next day, when Farage claimed that the Leave campaign's vision had come to pass "without a single bullet being fired."[52] Quite a few of us felt that his math was off by a tally of three.

In the days, weeks, and months that followed, anti-immigrant sentiment spiked. In the streets, people wore t-shirts reading "We Voted Leave, Now Get Out." Polish immigrants found their places of business spray-painted with the words "Go Home," and, in Cambridgeshire, leafleted with laminated cards (yes, laminated—the strangeness of that fact makes the cards all the more eerie) calling them "vermin."[53] Attacks on gay, lesbian, bisexual, and transgender people rose by 147% in the three months following the vote—a spike in hate-based crimes both higher than those faced by minority religious and ethnic groups and unprecedented in recent years.[54]

By summer, Farage had stepped down as head of UKIP and had gone on the campaign trail with Donald Trump. In a rally in Mississippi, he said,

Folks, the message is clear ... the parallels are there. There are millions of ordinary Americans who have been let down, who have had a bad time, who feel the political class in Washington is detached from them ... You can go out, you can beat the pollsters, you can beat the commentators, you can beat Washington.[55]

Unfortunately, Farage was right. And it's not just in the UK and US where we find those "parallels" that Farage spoke about. A large proportion of French voters recently rallied behind another far-right leader: Marine Le Pen, leader of the National Front.

Le Pen inherited her position as head of the National Front party from her father, Jean-Marie, an open anti-Semite who once remarked that the Nazi gas chambers that killed millions were just "a detail in the history of World War II."[56] While Le Pen has attempted to mop up the party's image by distancing it from her father's legacy, she's succeeded in doing so mostly by diverting racist fears away from Jews and toward Muslims; she has made comments—comments that led to a legal charge of inciting racial hatred— that Muslim people who pray in public are similar to the Nazi occupation of France.[57] She's also unafraid to take her father's financial backing despite the fact that he's been banned from the party since 2015; the elder Le Pen has claimed that he will contribute six million euro to his daughter's political causes.[58]

Like Trump and Farage, Marine Le Pen was once considered a noisy oddity on the fringes of the political process, and one polling too few votes to advance her beyond preliminary ballots. But not unlike the misleading polls on both Brexit and Trump, French polls failed to recognize how strongly Le Pen appealed to a world leaning precipitously to the right. Le Pen even positioned herself as part of a Trump-led movement, declaring that "Clearly Donald Trump's victory is an additional stone in the building of a new world, destined to replace the old one."[59]

The UK's Labour leader, Jeremy Corbyn (remember him?), had this to say about Le Pen:

> She uses this populism against minorities in order to get herself elected ... the reality is she does not have an economic answer to the problems faced by the left [behind] communities in France any more than UKIP has an economic answer to the left behind communities in Britain ... once you let this nasty thing out of the box called xenophobia and intolerance it's very hard to put it back.[60]

"Hard" is an understatement; the far right's hold on Europe isn't something that cleared up like a bad head cold upon Le Pen's loss to the centrist Emmanuel Macron. Le Pen galvanized a movement behind her— one that will continue to press for ever more discriminatory policies. That's proven true in the Netherlands, too, where racism drummed up by the Dutch Freedom Party's Geert Wilders thrives despite his unsuccessful bid to become prime minister. Wilders continues to rabble-rouse through his regular contributions to *Breitbart*, where he pens such ickily-titled articles as "We Must Preserve Western Identity" and "Let's Lock the Door to Islam," and his party's adherents haven't let up in their push to crush the country's Muslim population through such proposals as outlawing headscarves, closing mosques and schools, and banning the Koran.

Wilders himself (who, I can't refrain from pointing out, sports a perplexing hairstyle suggestive of melding Trump and Caesar Flickerman from the *Hunger Games* films, though the comedy of his hairdo belies the terrifying reality of his political views) has adopted such Trump tactics as taking to his personal Twitter account to make such statements as "NL has huge problem with Moroccans. To be silent about it is cowardly. 43% of Dutch want fewer Moroccans." He's made further anti-Moroccan remarks in his rallies, inciting crowds to chant "Fewer! Fewer!" with respect to how many Moroccan people should be allowed to live in the Netherlands. Wilders's discourse has been so offensive that he was put on trial to answer charges of hate speech, a crime in the Netherlands. But Wilders openly flouted the legal charges, refusing even to attend his own trial.[61] In early 2017, a three-person judiciary panel convicted Wilders of inciting discrimination. Yet to the surprise of onlookers around the globe, the panel declined to impose any penalty for the crime.[62]

The Dutch political sphere, one in which such legally prohibited remarks are taken so lightly, remains a frightening landscape for more liberal parties. One such example is the fledging political party Think, which attempts to provide a pro-immigrant, pro-multicultural political force that will, among other objectives, ban racist language from official use in the government and hold lawmakers accountable for hate speech. That all sounds like basic decency, but Sylvana Simons, a Dutch TV presenter turned Think politician who was running for a seat in parliament, became the focus of such intense racist abuse that it's painful even to summarize here. When Simons, a black woman born in Suriname, spoke publicly about the racist undertones of the Christmas holiday character Black Pete (often portrayed in festive parades by a white person in blackface), she found herself the subject of a viral video that superimposed her likeness on images of lynching victims. A television host suggested that Simons looked like a monkey, and played a sound clip of a gorilla to underscore his point.[63] The councilor in The Hague who reported the video to authorities called it "too disgusting for words," and the Think Party demanded security measures be put in place to ensure Simons's safety.[64]

What did Geert Wilders think of all this? He claimed that the only solution to the problem of racist abuse was for Simons to be "protected against herself and her party (Think) to be disbanded." It's worth noting that Wilders, because of his anti-Islam remarks throughout his political career, has been under special, government-supported protection designed to ensure his personal safety for the past decade.[65] In the wake of the racist abuse, Simons left the Think party, saying that it had done to little to protect her, and formed the new party Artikel 1.[66]

It's been equally hard to put that xenophobia and intolerance that Corbyn mentioned back in the box elsewhere in Europe; in Hungary, the Jobbik party—which has proposed, among other alarming changes to law, prison terms of up to eight years for the crime of being gay—will seek to become the governing party of the nation by 2018.[67] Should Jobbik succeed, it will replace the ruling right-wing party, Fidesz, which itself is no angelic presence in Europe; Fidesz recently sponsored a parliamentary bill to ban migrants from the country, and has employed such methods as installing razor-wire fences at its borders to keep refugees from entering.[68]

Outside the EU, unaffiliated states are swinging to the right as well.

Sweden's anti-immigrant party, The Sweden Democrats (with its white-supremacist and neo-Nazi roots[69]), won 13% of the vote in the country's 2014 election. Finland, Denmark, and even Switzerland have seen significant gains for far-right parties over the past decade.[70]

With EU member states sliding so far to the right, and with EU Chancellor Angela Merkel (whose recent calls for bans on Muslim women wearing full-face veils in Germany have raised serious questions about her commitment to a progressive and inclusive Europe[71]) up for an uncertain reelection bid, many have begun to fear that the EU's stabilizing presence will crumble. Such an outcome would have far-reaching consequences, including the effective halting of the free movement of people across all European borders. It could also have disastrous consequences for disabled people—a group that, both here in the US and in Europe, needs perhaps the most legal safeguards, though it receives the least.

Already, the UK is no welcoming place for disabled residents, who face increasing pushback against their right to access public space. Just this past January, Anne Wafula-Strike, a UK paralympian whose contributions to sports in the British Empire earned her the distinction of MBE (a Member of the Most Excellent Order of the British Empire—Americans can think of this as somewhere in the general zip code of knighthood) was subjected to a humiliating ordeal on a long-haul train. Wafula-Strike was well into her journey home from a meeting of the UK Athletics Board when she was informed that the train she was riding had no functional disabled bathrooms (this despite the fact that riders needing accommodations must prebook their journeys to alert staff to their needs). Without appropriate facilities or even assistance to an accessible bathroom at the next train station, Wafula-Strike was forced to urinate in her clothes. She was offered some free tickets by the rail company by way of an "apology."[72]

Around the same time, UK resident Doug Paulley wrapped up a multi-year legal battle for bus access—one that he and activist groups fought all the way through the Supreme Court. In 2012, Paulley was denied access to a bus because a mother refused to move her sleeping infant's stroller out of the zone reserved for disabled transit users, leaving Paulley, a wheelchair user, stranded at the curb. The absurdity of having to take such a claim—a claim that disabled people should have priority access to disabled spaces—to the highest court of law is one that a nonplussed Paulley summed up like so: "Who would have thought that five years on I would still being discussing the day I had that problem going across to see my parents for lunch?"[73]

Despite the Court's ruling in Paulley's favor, just weeks later, some bus drivers were openly flouting their responsibilities to disabled riders. Wakefield resident Kristy Shepherd was denied entry to a bus because—you guessed it—a parent with a stroller had chosen to occupy the area reserved for wheelchair access. Shepherd demanded access (and the parent agreed to move to the empty stroller-priority space of the bus to allow room for her), but the driver insisted that he would not allow Shepherd on. Instead, he asked passengers to disembark and reprimand Shepherd, saying that it was her fault that the bus journey couldn't continue on to its destination. The other passengers were all too willing to comply, and stepped off the bus to give Shepherd a lecture on her selfishness.[74]

If it weren't bad enough that disabled residents are increasingly squeezed out of public space, a recent double-down on austerity measures means that disabled people who now live independently may be forcibly institutionalized. The activist group Disability United recently blew the whistle on England's National Health Service for its plans to warehouse up to 13,000 British residents unless those individuals raise the money to pay for continued in-home care.[75] Beyond the obvious injustice of shaking down disabled people, their families, and their communities for cash under a socialized system that purportedly guarantees free and equal care for all, the move is tantamount to threatening patients with violence; care homes in the UK are notorious for mistreating those forced to live in them. The innocuously-named Winterbourne View, to give just one example, was the site of such extraordinary patient mistreatment that, after an undercover BBC investigative report, six workers were tried and sentenced for abuse and neglect. I could recount here the scores of injustices that patients faced in Winterbourne View, but a single detail perhaps sums it up best: one worker reportedly enjoyed pretending to be a Nazi soldier and put on a German accent while beating the residents.[76]

The situation doesn't stand to get any better in a post-Brexit society. The EU has been one of the greatest drivers of legislation to protect people with disabilities from abuse, discrimination, and limited access throughout Europe; without the EU's center of legal gravity surrounding disability, residents face growing uncertainties about their basic rights and inclusion in society. Once the UK finally severs its ties with EU, citizens could very well see rollbacks of EU-constituted disability rights laws, such as the Framework Directive for Equal Treatment in Employment in Occupation, which prevents employment discrimination. Prior to the EU's intervention, the UK held a smattering of anti-discrimination laws, but those laws allowed small companies—ones with 20 employees or fewer—

to discriminate against disabled employees without repercussions. The EU further legislated that member states cannot discriminate against employees due to their relationships with disabled people—no one could be fired or harassed in the workplace because of a need to care for a disabled child or spouse.[77]

Even if the UK doesn't rescind the current EU legislation—though there is no reason to believe that it will retain any EU laws—disabled people in the UK will certainly miss out on newly proposed EU legislation that will, when ratified, improve access to public buildings, transport, banking, and digital services across all member states.[78]

Should the EU face dissolution (a scenario that seems mercifully less likely in light of a Le Pen rout, though euroskepticism continues to grow among populist bases), all European residents could see further setbacks to disability rights. The EU-ratified Convention on the Rights of Persons with Disabilities, the first and only international agreement designed specifically to uphold the rights of disabled people, legally binds member states not only to ensure non-discrimination policies, but also to provide the support and services that disabled people need in order to fully participate in and contribute to society.[79] Among its many provisions, the Convention obligates member states to invest in assistive technologies, mobility aids, and accessible information, and to eliminate discriminatory policies in public and private enterprises.[80] Without the EU as a watchdog, individual nations (including a freshly Brexited UK) will have no oversight holding them to their legal obligations.

I once knew a man who spent no small amount of time complaining about the city of Fresno. Regardless of what challenges the nation faced, he would allow nothing to compete with his idea of his hometown's awfulness. If there was a spate of gun crime in Chicago, surely it couldn't match the level of violence in Fresno. If traffic clogged the Los Angeles freeways, at least it wasn't as bad as it was in Fresno. If a wildfire broke out and filled the skies over Oklahoma with smoke, the air was still dirtier in Fresno. If unemployment was high in the Rust Belt, it wasn't as high as it was in Fresno.

Today, many years on, he's still living in Fresno and complaining about his city at every opportunity. Yet he hasn't made any efforts to contribute something positive to his community or to help solve any of the many ills he thinks he's identified. Instead, he plans to one day move away.

He may have a bizarre fixation on the downsides of a perfectly nice city in central California, but he's unfortunately not so different from the rest of us Americans.

We have a tendency, fostered from an early age, to view the US as unique. When we've looked at our nation as uniquely good or even uniquely qualified to lead the world, that attitude has led us to disastrous foreign intervention, to willful injustice and inequality at home, and to the waving around of the name of God as though he personally endorsed the worst and most unethical of our policies and leaders. Yet there exists an equally unhelpful B-side to the notion that America is special: when our national attitude slides toward intolerance and hatred, we assume that we're alone in our sorrow and fear. We nurture the idea that our position—and our ability to do anything about it—is worse than it is anywhere else in the global community. In our grief over our present and concern for our future, we give ourselves the luxury of ignoring the burdens carried by the rest of the world. It's that very ignorance that makes us want to seek a safe haven that's never existed, and we become that old man ranting about Fresno from his air-conditioned living room.

The fact that our political and social climate is just one part of a broader global shift may feel, at first, like a comfort. We all know the adage about misery and company. We'd be merely indulging ourselves if we didn't turn that commiseration into action; instead of looking toward the rest of the world for shelter, perhaps we Americans might try to learn from the examples all around us. How were figures like Le Pen and Wilders discredited among enough voters to ensure their election-night losses? Will stabilizing political forces manage to check their continued popular appeal? Which tactics work and which fail in resisting demagoguery? What initiatives actually help vulnerable populations, and which take unintended tolls on the groups they are designed to safeguard? How can those who share goals work together despite ideological differences? What social patterns can we identify and learn from as we combat hate and intolerance?

It's tempting to say that it's never been more important to resist hopelessness and instead focus on action—putting our resources where they will have a cumulative, positive effect on our world. But in truth, it's always been this important to turn toward our responsibilities as human beings. Maybe now we're simply reaping the consequences of our long inaction.

LOSS REPORT

Four days before I left the United Kingdom for good, I was out for a final London dinner with colleagues. It was a celebratory gathering, marking the end of a work-heavy publication season and the upcoming launch of some gorgeous books the next day—much better than a sad and sorry goodbye dinner.

We ate too much butter chicken for waistband comfort and drank too much beer for a work night at the family-owned restaurant on the Boundary Road, but I didn't know how many months or even years would pass before I saw these people again. As the late night slid toward early morning, I poked at the saucy remainder on my plate and ignored the clock as it wound toward the last train of the night.

It was still warm when it was time to make my way back to the flat where I'd been living alone for the past six weeks (my husband was back in the US, settling into his new, post-Brexit job while I wrang out the last days of my UK visa). I walked in my shirtsleeves through the quiet streets of St. John's Wood toward the tube station, strolling past the enormous mansions and multi-million-pound flats, navigating among the roots of trees dropping early leaves on sports cars. The neighborhood is one of the poshest spots in London, though it's one not too many Americans would know by its name. Most anyone in the world, though, would recognize the place the moment they saw the crosswalk immortalized on The Beatles' *Abbey Road* album.

For as long as I'd been living in London, in my more down-to-earth neighborhood to the north, I'd intended to swing by and get a good photo of that crossing. I'd wanted to send a picture to my father. But it was too dark now.

When I was growing up, the house was never quiet. It wasn't just that there were always screaming kids around—first my sister and me and then my kid brothers—but also the fact that there was never a time when my parents didn't have music playing.

If my mom had her way, what came over our stereo would have been all John Denver, Neil Diamond, and Barry Manilow (with a peppering of Abba for a little pick-me-up). My father would have preferred Crosby, Stills & Nash, the Allman Brothers, and Neil Young. The one musical act they could agree on was The Beatles.

Even so, she was a McCartney fan, and devoured those poppier songs about wanting to hold hands or feeling fine while he liked Lennon and the Sergeant Pepper years, complete with walrus.

As for me, I'd later become a George Harrison kind of girl, preferring the weeping guitar and the sun coming out to the big sonic wall of "Hey Jude." But as a kid, I'd bop around the house in our musical demilitarized zone that fell somewhere around the *Rubber Soul* era, singing about the Nowhere Man and how good Norwegian wood was in the room of a girl who once had Lennon. And, of course I had the right surrealistic frame of childhood mind to appreciate, once we'd burned our way through that record and onto *Revolver,* the idea of living in a submarine with a large colony of other people.

Later, as a teenager in the '90s, the rest of my musical tastes ran toward bands like The Smashing Pumpkins and Radiohead and away from those of my parents, but we could still agree on The Beatles. I was a *White Album* fan by then, but that was as far as I was willing to rebel against the group positivity we all held for one band. When the rediscovered "Free as a Bird" single was finally released in 1995, we even sat down—in a rare moment of joint family activity—to watch the music video when it debuted on VH1.

As the years moved on and my parents slid deeper into the far-right politics and increasingly fringe religious beliefs that I would never share nor even pretend to understand, here in this music was one thing we could hold in common. We had this, even if we had nothing else.

I got on what may have been the last Bakerloo line train of the night and settled back onto the scarred upholstery. I pulled out my phone as I always do on the Tube, popping in my earbuds to ward off the conversation of strange men who'd just left the pub. I clicked open a music app to keep me occupied for the ride home.

Just as the ancient train car screamed and jounced its way out of the station and beyond the reach of the wifi signal, I flipped my email open— another train reflex of mine—and saw that I had one new message. It was from my mother.

The message said that, after thirty-seven years, my father had walked out.

Two days later the movers—"removals men," as the British have it—were due at my flat to catalogue and label all of my possessions. I'd been up until four the night before, having played the composed editor at the book launch, then put back more wine than necessary at the after event. Finally, in the early hours, I began to pack up my home.

I'd delayed boxing up my belongings and sorting through my things; I wasn't ready to leave England, and I'd been trying to squeeze out the last enjoyment from my time there, the time before the EU Referendum squeezed us foreigners out amid the plummeting currency, the cries of "Britain first," and the many months of political uncertainty. But I paid for my procrastination—packing up was a chore, but moving always is. Now that I was out of time, it wasn't the manual labor but the taking apart of our home that we'd worked so hard to make that grated at me. Preparing to leave our life in England felt too emotionally tied up in the breakdown of my family a continent away.

When the movers finally came, they picked through the accumulations of my life and slapped stickers on the boxes that would carry my shoes and dishes and books and paintings over the ocean. Normally, I'd have been horrified as they tossed my novels into boxes without concern for case-bound corners of rare editions, or by the seemingly Dada manner in which they mixed clothing with dishes with shampoos with throw pillows in giant, unwieldy boxes. But in my exhaustion, I couldn't find it in me to care.

I stepped around the men as they worked, trying to stay out of their way. I took extra care not to hook a toe on the mess of power cords that I'd unplugged from walls and stashed in the corner, or to tangle with the rolled-up rug that I'd leaned upright in the hall. The doctor treating my bone loss had recently given me a stern warning about tripping and falling. The steroid drug treatment that had kept me alive for the past few years had come at a cost to my bones, a cost that had grown so expensive as to become full-blown osteoporosis by the time I was 33. She wanted me to remember that it wouldn't take a bus crash or a train derailment to injure me—I could grind down my bones with any misstep on the sloping floors of my old Victorian apartment. She gave me her talk about avoiding what she called "the stupid stuff": twisting an ankle in high heels, catching a toe on a tree root in the park, losing my balance while reaching for a high shelf. Add enough of that stupid stuff together and I'd be well on my way to badly broken.

The movers handed me stacks of documents printed on triplicate, asking me to tick off boxes and to initial dozens of pages saying that all was well and that everything was accounted for. I scribbled a rough approximation of my signature and stuffed the pink and yellow pages into my bag. I didn't bother to read them—with my right hand, I was busy texting my mother 4,800 miles and an eight-hour time difference away.

My mother sketched for me the broad outlines of the past few months. It was as tawdry and tired as the plot of a bad film. There was my father's mid-life crisis, the sudden desire to play cover songs in local bars. The attentions of the local divorcees. The casting about for such a divorcee who looked young enough in the half-light and scrim of Pabst Blue Ribbon until he finally found a taker. The moving out from, the moving in with.

I stood in my kitchen, stunned as men walked from my flat, carrying the contents of my life out to the street in every armload.

With each new message that floated onto my iPhone screen in a cheerfully shaped text bubble, the story grew more pathetic—it was such a vulgar end to a marriage and a family. My father hadn't even told me that story himself. He let that fall to my mother, the person whose life he'd just upended.

Had I been able to eat for the past few days, I'd likely have vomited; my guts twisted with that same sick feeling I'd had every Sunday when belted into the back of the family station wagon, speeding to church along winding back roads. There was no week of my childhood that my father didn't drag us to that storefront church to hear a semiliterate pastor—one who didn't know the word "wrath"—preach about "the raft of God." Some Sundays, he made me stand on the side of the road, breathing in car exhaust and holding an "abortion is murder" poster that was bigger than I was as my church dress flapped in the hot California air. On weeknights, when the evening news came on, he'd mutter "feminazi" or "grow some hair" over whatever Janet Reno or Hillary Clinton had to say on screen. "This women's lib thing has gone too far," he'd say, just loudly enough that I couldn't hear those women speak. After meals, he'd tell me how fat I'd get if I kept on eating the way I did. There were so many years of it—so much *stupid stuff* that I couldn't fight against as a kid. I thought I'd put it all down, stacked it up in the long hall of my childhood as I walked into adult life on my own. But in truth, it was this stupid stuff that I'd been tripping on and stumbling over for years. It had left me ready to break now, all the way down to the marrow.

.*. *.* .*.

It's not news that we human beings have a tendency to protest too much—to hold forth the most passionately on what we're the least certain about. Contested leaders cite their "mandates" from the people, those who can't grasp science rely on "faith," and my father talked about "the family."

It wasn't unusual to hear him insist that my mom, my siblings, and I were the most important feature of his life, but these speeches always came with the air of a man talking to himself, reconciling his own mind to something none of us knew to be true. Of course, I wanted to believe him—in the way that any daughter wants to believe that she's loved, that she is irreplaceable and necessary—yet I put the most weight on the way my father looked at me when he didn't think I was watching. He'd eye me with a slightly perplexed tilt of his head and a look that suggested he couldn't quite remember where I'd come from, or why I was here.

The right-wing *Focus on the Family* magazines with which he littered the coffee table only underscored my suspicions. If the family was such a good thing, why would we need a magazine to tell us how to appreciate it? Who were we trying to convince?

I myself had decided early on that "the family" wasn't something I wanted to focus on, but something I'd have to endure. For years, I kept quiet when he tossed the phrase "when you have kids of your own" into conversation. I knew better than to voice contrary opinions—I was already on notice for being unpleasant, rude, disrespectful, unladylike. But as a teenager, when I was as prone to rebellion as I was going to get, I told my father, "I don't *want* to have kids of my own."

"You'll change your mind," he said.

I never did.

In the days, weeks, and months after my father's walking out, I waited for a phone call: the one in which he would explain himself, or make even the most half-hearted defense of his choices.

It never came.

I began to understand: he was the one who'd changed his mind.

A month after I left England, I stood in the kitchen in my new home in New Jersey, stirring the chili I was making in the one pot I had, using the one spoon I had, so that my husband and I could eat our dinner from the two bowls I'd flown to the US in my suitcase. We'd eat, as we had for the past few weeks, while sitting with our legs folded beneath us.

121

My back ached, and sitting on floor didn't help. I'd lost about an inch of my spine in the last two years, my vertebrae compacting and shrinking into themselves as bone crumbled into other bone. I twisted to pop my lower spine for a momentary relief, though every time I did, I worried that I might be breaking myself down more and more.

I comforted myself that we wouldn't have to sit on the floor much longer; the next morning, a moving truck would carry our shipment to our driveway. A different crew of workmen would unload our crates, and I'd be reunited with some of my earthly goods. I looked forward to feeling like someone who had an address of her own rather than like a squatter hiding out in an empty house. I might even be able, if I could find my speakers somewhere in the bottom of a box, to listen to some music as I unpacked.

My husband's cell phone scuttled and buzzed across the cardboard box that we were using as a table. Over the kitchen fan's drone, I could hear him answer the call in his extra-friendly phone voice—a voice that, for some reason, always sounds higher than his natural speech. It was the movers, I imagined, ringing us to confirm their delivery time.

I was ladling our dinner into our bowls as well as I could with my flat, wooden spoon when I heard him say, "Oh, God." His voice had dropped by an octave.

I turned down the flame on the range and walked out to where he stood in the living room, one hand beneath the dripping, saucy spoon I was still holding in the other.

I gave him the raised-eyebrow that asked, "What's up?"

Still listening to the voice on the other end of the line, he mouthed the word "fire."

In a stockyard somewhere in Maryland, the truck carrying our earthly goods and those of at least four other families had exploded into flames. No one could tell us what had happened, or whether the catalyst had been a malfunction of the truck, a collision, or even something as foolish as the smolder of a lithium battery that should never have been transported by truck to begin with.

What the moving company could tell us, however, was that the fire began toward the back of the shipping container. It burned its way first through one person's boxes, then consumed another's and another's until it finally reached the front of the truck and scorched through ours. They planned to take our things to a salvage site in Virginia and pick through what remained.

Maybe we'd get lucky, the customer service rep on the other end of the line told us. It might just be a bit of smoke damage here, some water marks there. It wasn't the end of the world; we might not lose everything.

The day after my seventeenth birthday, my parents moved us out of our house in Fresno, California, drove us and all of our belongings to my grandparents' home in the hills, and waited for the apocalypse.

As the year 2000 approached, most educated people agreed that the so-called "Y2K Bug" wouldn't have many wide-spread effects. A few fringe Christians like my parents—people for whom Pat Robertson's *The 700 Club* was the primary news source and who would have shelved their copies of Hal Lindsey's *Apocalypse Code* under nonfiction—couldn't wait for "the end times" to arrive. The close of the millennium was the best shot they'd ever had at Armageddon.

I suppose it was the very lack of technological progress evident in our home that allowed my parents such credence in the "bug" to begin with; in 1999, we didn't have an internet connection, much less a functional computer or, God forbid, a printer (I was still writing my high school papers on an IBM typewriter and hoping not to run out of black ribbon or correction fluid around the time my midterm papers were due). Perhaps it was precisely because they were so far removed from technology that my parents felt that they knew what was "really going on."

What would come for humanity in January, they said, wouldn't be some mere inconveniences with those Gateway home computers that came from massive, Holstein-patterned boxes. The "bug" would fry PCs, yes, but it would next collapse the power grid. Sewers, unable to keep a flow of water moving without access to power, would back up and fill both homes and city streets with human waste. People would grow sick and die. That's when martial law would commence.

Luckily for us, they believed, we wouldn't be around to see it. We'd be far off in the hills, tilling the soil and growing crops on the hillside dust and hardpan that had so far sustained nothing but ancient oak trees. They'd spent the past year accumulating viable wheat in ten-gallon buckets, the stump-like drums of grain lining the crawl space beneath the house like the remains of a clear-cut forest.

To supplement the wheat stores, they bought peaches, canned in heavy syrup, or that viscous fruit cocktail studded with nuclear-pink cherries. For protein, there was preserved meat, chunky with bones and gristle. That would carry everyone over, my parents said, until we learned to hunt. What, exactly, we would hunt wasn't clear, but my father would walk off into the hills with his unlicensed and unregistered handgun—the one he stored in a mailing envelope on top of a dresser—and unload rounds at unsuspecting squirrels and gophers.

There weren't enough beds in my grandparents' house for me to have one that winter. The twin bed I'd slept on throughout my childhood was either lost in the shuffle or deemed unnecessary for the end times, though no one ever told me which. For a few nights, my grandparents let me sleep in their truck camper, but it was far too expensive, they told me, to keep filling the little propane heater that kept me warm. I'd have to move into the living room and take the couch.

There weren't any blankets this time—those stayed with the camper. But I found an old sleeping bag in a cobwebbed corner of the garage and shook it clear of bugs and twigs for me. I laid it out on the lumpy couch next to the television where my toddler brothers watched *Barney and Friends* on a ceaseless loop. For privacy and for darkness enough to sleep, I had a pillow I could toss over my face. The wood stove across from me burned the air dry, and I'd wake with the skin around my eyes and mouth cracked and bleeding.

I stayed up as late as I could in the frozen winter nights. I dragged my school books, wire-ringed notepads, and homework to an outbuilding at the base of the hill. I tried to ignore the yellow eyes of coyotes that followed me from the roadside as I walked. Inside the structure, all-weather carpet nubbed the floor, and the fat spiders and tiny scorpions darted from my flashlight's beam, but the building had a functional heater fitted in the wall, and nobody—yet—had forbidden me to use it. I'd fire up the unit and press my mittened hands against the grill until my fingers had sensation enough to grab a pen. I sat on the floor and worked, my own spine and the spines of my cracked-open books protesting less and less as the months went on.

In that quiet of the night hours, while my father waited for the world to end, I learned the long and labor-intensive practice of hope: I studied for my honors courses and my advanced placement exams, lighting my work with a flashlight. I read the copy of *Siddhartha* that I hid from my parents lest one throw it out for being "pagan." I clouted out my college application essays on my typewriter and hand-addressed the manila envelopes in which I'd mail them off. I read books that hadn't been assigned to me. I wrote bad poems. I imagined a future beyond 1999. While my father played the survivalist, I taught myself how to survive.

On New Year's Eve, the apocalypse didn't come the way my parents had hoped; there was no pale horse and no plague swept the continents. When the apocalypse came, it sounded like the 150 slot machines in Delaware that had stopped spinning their fruit wheels at midnight. It sounded like a bus ticket machine in Australia that couldn't validate passenger fares for a few hours, and like an incorrect weather forecast that was aired on French TV. It sounded like my grandparents' bathtub down the hall still filling with emergency drinking water as midnight rolled across our time zone. It sounded like my headphones blaring out the absurd lyrics to "I Am The Walrus" where I lay in my sleeping bag, draining my double-A batteries to drown out my family's disappointment at the world's grinding on.

After the moving company delivered news of the fire, my husband and I drove to the local IKEA and picked out a bed. We'd come to a life stage at which we could likely have afforded something a notch above the endless string of Malms that would splinter and creak, but when the grown-up furniture stores gave us months-long wait times for bed frames, I realized how eager I was to get off the floor. I'd begun to feel displaced in our own empty house, and the lack of a real bed as we waited for news of our scorched possessions only recalled that bleak winter in the California hills.

In the IKEA show room, we wrote down the aisle and bin numbers of the least offensive frame, then wandered through a row of closet cabinets and thought about the way we'd organize what items might return to us one day from that warehouse in Virginia.

All around us couples grumbled at one another with that unique, IKEA-induced combination of low blood sugar, mismatched personal tastes, and controversy over room dimensions. Kids howled as parents pulled them off displays they were scaling like so many feral cats. Across the room was a product I'd read about in the paper: a vast and homely cabinet measuring seven feet in height that was so miserable to assemble that it had been nicknamed "The Divorcemaker." Over the years, it had been our running (if grim) joke that any marriage and family therapist in want of clientele should wander the IKEA floors and hand out business cards at random.

That joke didn't seem so funny any longer as the series of text messages from my mother pinged away inside my jeans pocket.

.*. *.* .*.

It would be a month before the moving company finished sorting through our ruin. When they were confident that they'd found all that remained of our belongings, they sent us an email with the subject line "Davio: Loss Report."

Attached was a string of photos of what the salvage crew had managed to pull from the truck. Here was our dining room table, gouged by a firefighter's ax. And here a torched box filled with an unidentifiable mess that might have been dishes at some point, though it was impossible to tell from the photos taken in such poor light. Many of our things, torched beyond saving, had never been identified at all.

Interspersed with the crime-scene-like shots of our belongings were objects we didn't recognize—strange items belonging to some other family. They were lawn ornaments, mostly, and Christmas décor. In the middle of one up-ended box was a scorched Halloween costume—a child-sized witch's outfit. The pointed black hat lay deflated in the bottom of the cardboard box. It looked to me as though the little girl who'd worn it had burned down to nothing.

Not long after, the moving company stopped responding to our emails asking when the insurance check would finally arrive. While my husband did what most people would do—got angry, left increasingly stern voice messages, and demanded that the company expedite our claim—I didn't believe the movers would ever call, just as I knew that my father wouldn't. I've been trained my whole life for letdown.

The week of Christmas I lay on the table under the DEXA machine in the hospital's imaging center. The device whirred above me as the tech strapped my feet to the plastic block that would hold them in place for the high-resolution X-rays. The resulting images would measure how much more of my bone had wasted away this year. The question wasn't whether my bones had gotten worse—the question was merely how bad it was this time—how much unseen damage had been done over the year.

The tech went over my patient questionnaire, confirming that no, I hadn't taken any calcium pills that morning, and, no, there wasn't any possibility that I was pregnant. She scanned the list of my medications and stopped when she came to the osteoporosis drugs.

"You're taking bisphosphonates? At your age?"

It's never a comfort to be an outlier, a never-seen-one-of-these-before. "I have osteoporosis," I told her. "I've lost a lot of bone already."

The machine whirred and hummed as it warmed up, drowning out the last part of that sentence. It sounded as though I'd said only *I've lost a lot.*

When the insurance check came, its envelope fell through the front door mail slot with an unceremonious plunk. I opened the envelope, detached the check from its lengthy stub, and held it for a moment, unprepared for the fact of its existence. I left it on the kitchen counter for a day, then two days, three.

It had been many weeks of my husband's sending off increasingly harsh emails with vague threats of legal action before the movers told us that we could have either our insurance money or what remained of our salvaged goods in that warehouse in Virginia—not both. At first, I couldn't understand the pettiness of such an arrangement, or why they'd given us all those images of our burnt and sorry stuff to sort through if it would never be returned to us in the first place. I began to suspect that someone in the warehouse had misplaced those last boxes belonging to us, tossed them out into the back dumpster for hauling off to the landfill.

What I'd been waiting to return to me—the old snapshots, the fake and glittery 60s Christmas tree, my warm blankets, my melted record collection with its copies of *Abbey Road, Sergeant Pepper* and all—was no doubt already buried under garbage, already being picked over by crows hopping along in the rot. As ugly as that thought was, I didn't mind it so much; I had no more desire to pick through the charred wreckage of my life. All the lost things I'd hoped would come back to me—just as I'd hoped my father might one day come back to me—they were long gone. Gone as the bone washed out of my spine.

But here on my kitchen counter, the insurance check waited for me. It waited the way my books, my college applications, and my bad poems had all waited in the coldest winter of my life. It was a reminder of the hope I'd taught myself: maybe this wasn't the end of the world. Maybe I wouldn't lose everything.

I cashed the check.

ACKNOWLEDGMENTS

Essays in this collection have previously appeared, sometimes in slightly different forms, in *The Rumpus, The Nervous Breakdown, The Butter,* and *Change Seven Magazine,* and I want to extend heartfelt thanks to the editors who shaped them (and me) along the way: Roxane Gay, Erika Kleinman, Nicole Chung, Sheryl Monks, and Antonios Maltezos. You helped me find my voice.

I'm also deeply in debt to the incredible women who gave me their time, feedback, and support throughout the writing of this book: Tanya Chernov Smith, Jeannine Hall Gailey, Yi Shun Lai, and the members of Book Lift and MyWags.

I'm grateful to Peter, whose belief in my writing often exceeds my own, and whose support and encouragement are the great constants of my life.

Finally, my deep thanks go to Raymond Luczak, who singlehandedly made this book possible. Thank you for the gift of your work.

ABOUT THE AUTHOR

Kelly Davio is the Poetry Editor of *Tahoma Literary Review* and the author of the poetry collections *Burn This House* (2013) and *The Book of the Unreal Woman* (forthcoming, 2018). While living in England, she was an editor with Eyewear Publishing. Previously, she spent many years teaching English as a Second Language to secondary students in Seattle. Today she lives and writes in New Jersey.

ENDNOTES

1   Katherine Bindley. "Leggings Banned As Pants: Backlash Over Girls' Dress Code At Kenilworth Junior High." *Huffington Post*. Apr. 9, 2013.
2   Naomi S. Baron. "The case against e-readers: why reading paper books is better for your mind." *The Washington Post*. Jan. 12, 2015.
3   Amy Kraft. "Books vs. ebooks: The science behind the best way to read." *CBS News*. Dec. 14, 2015.
4   "Subminimum Wage." *United States Department of Labor*. https://www.dol.gov/general/topic/wages/subminimumwage
5   Kim Painter and Nanci Hellmich. "Amelia Rivera gets kidney after transplant debate." *USA Today*. Jul. 30, 2013.
6   "'Compassionate homicide': The law and Robert Latimer." *CBC News*. Dec. 6, 2010.
7   John Allen Paulus. "The Odds Are You're Innumerate." *The New York Times*. Jan. 1, 1989.
8   Wallace Stevens. "A Rabbit as King of the Ghosts." *Poetryfoundation.org*. https://www.poetryfoundation.org/poetrymagazine/poems/detail/21816
9   Chris Johnston. "Britain's new foreign secretary Boris Johnson: a career of insults and gaffes." *The Guardian*. Jul. 13, 2016.
10   Jordan Weissmann. "The Campaign Lie That's Coming Back to Haunt Brexit Supporters." *Slate*. Jun. 27, 2016.
11   Andrew Griffin. "Brexit: Vote Leave wipes NHS £350m claim and rest of its website after EU referendum." *Independent*. Jun. 27, 2016.
12   Denis Campbell. "BMA: Theresa May lacks understanding about seriousness of NHS crisis." *The Guardian*. Oct. 15, 2016.
13   Laura Donnelly and Henry Bodkin. "NHS crisis plan to cancel operations and appointments as winter draws in." *The Telegraph*. Aug. 21, 2016.
14   Press Association. "Norovirus cases in England at highest level in five years." *The Guardian*. Dec. 30, 2016.
15   Toby Helm. "Number of urgent operations cancelled in England hits record high." *The Guardian*. Dec. 24, 2016.
16   Denis Campbell and Anna Bawden. "A&E, cancer and maternity units to close in major NHS overhaul." *The Guardian*. Nov. 18, 2016.
17   Nicola Harley. "NHS denies Red Cross claims there is a 'humanitarian crisis' in UK hospitals." *The Telegraph*. Jan. 7, 2017.

18 "'That' bus gets a Greenpeace makeover to replace 'lies' with 10,000 questions for the new government." *ITV*. Jul. 18, 2016.

19 Sarah Boseley. "Breast cancer drug rejected for NHS use on cost-benefit grounds." *The Guardian*. Dec. 28, 2016.

20 Frances Perraudin. "AA Gill's final column says NHS could not give him new cancer treatment." *The Guardian*. Dec. 11, 2016.

21 AA Gill. "More life with your kids, more life with your friends, more life spent on earth—but only if you pay." *The Times*. Dec. 11, 2016.

22 Asa Bennet. "Junior doctors strike: why are they taking action and how will it affect you?" *The Telegraph*. Apr. 6, 2016.

23 British Medical Association. Press release: "Junior doctors reject proposed contract." Jul. 5, 2016. www.bma.org.uk

24 Deborah Orr. "So, junior doctors, what exactly is it you're striking for?" *The Guardian*. Sep. 2, 2016.

25 Shane Croucher. "Jeremy Hunt: Should British workers work harder like the Chinese and Americans?" *International Business Times*. Oct. 6, 2015.

26 Nick Triggle. "Junior doctors' strike: Second all-out stoppage hits NHS." *BBC News*. Apr. 27, 2016.

27 Sarah Boseley and Matthew Weaver. "Junior doctors' row: BMA announces more five-day strikes." *The Guardian*. Sep. 1, 2016.

28 Supra note 16.

29 Haroon Siddique. "NHS hospital waiting time figures worst in seven years." *The Guardian*. Apr. 9, 2015.

30 Colin Yeo. "Comprehensive Sickness Insurance: what is it, and who needs it?" *Freemovement.org.uk*. Jul. 18, 2016.

31 Supra note 18.

32 Denis Campbell. "Ban NHS doctors from private work, hospital consultant says." *The Guardian*. May 5, 2016.

33 Kailash Chand. "2016 was the worst year in NHS history—we must fight for its survival." *The Guardian*. Jan. 4, 2017.

34 Haroon Siddique and Rowena Mason. "PM under fire for saying foreign doctors are in UK only for 'interim period.'" *The Guardian*. Oct. 4, 2016.

35 Aisha Harris. "The *Empire* Finale Delivered a 'Splash, Punch' to the Senses." *Slate*. Mar. 19, 2015.

36 Stacey Wade. "Static/Major." You Tube. Aug. 23, 3009.

37 Phillip M. Bailey. "Static star." *Leo Weekly*. Feb. 25, 2009.

38 Catherine Shoard. "The Theory of Everything review: Hawking's story packs powerful punch." *The Guardian*. Sep. 7, 2014.

39 "Daniel Radcliffe's Cripple of Inishmaan wows Broadway Critics." *BBC News*. Apr. 21, 2014.

40 Allan V. Horowitz. "How an Age of Anxiety Became an Age of Depression." *Millbank Quarterly*. 2010; 88(1): 112–138.

41 Shadia Kawa and James Giordano. "A brief historicity of the Diagnostic and Statistical Manual of Mental Disorders: Issues and implications for the future of psychiatric canon and practice." *Philosophy, Ethics, and Humanities in Medicine: PEHM.* 2012; 10.1186/1747-5341-7-2.

42 Richard Gallagher. "As a psychiatrist, I diagnose mental illness. Also, I help spot demonic possession." *The Washington Post.* Jul. 1, 2016.

43 "Crucified nun dies in 'exorcism.'" *BBC News.* Jun. 18, 2005.

44 John Kabat-Zinn. *Coming to Our Senses.* Hachette Books, 2005.

45 Ben Westcott. "Brexit leader Nigel Farage calls Obama a loathsome creature." *CNN Politics.* Nov. 11, 2016.

46 Rowena Mason. "Nigel Farage accuses Muslims in UK of 'split loyalties.'" *The Guardian.* Nov. 16, 2015.

47 Ewan Palmer. "Nigel Farage resigns: Most infamous quotes from outgoing UKIP leader." *International Business Times.* Jul. 4, 2016.

48 Josh Lowe. "Brexit: UKIP launches 'Breaking Point' Immigration Poster." *Newsweek.* Jun. 16, 2016.

49 Heather Steward and Rowena Mason. "Nigel Farage's anti-migrant poster reported to police." *The Guardian.* Jun. 16, 2016.

50 Ishaan Tharoor. "Brexit leader said victory came without a bullet being fired. He seems to have forgotten Jo Cox." *The Washington Post.* Jun. 24, 2016.

51 "Labour MP Jo Cox 'murdered for political cause.'" *BBC News.* Nov. 14, 2016.

52 Supra note 50.

53 "Anti-Polish cards in Huntingdon after EU referendum." *BBC News.* Jun. 26, 2016.

54 Mark Townsend. "Homophobic attacks in UK rose 147% in three months after Brexit vote." *The Guardian.* Oct. 8, 2016.

55 Roger Cohen. "The Trump-Farage Road Show." *The New York Times.* Aug. 29, 2016.

56 Cecile Alduy. "The Devil's Daughter." *The Atlantic.* Oct. 2013.

57 "France's Le Pen on trial over Muslim comments." *Aljazeera.* Oct. 20, 2015.

58 Nicholas Vinocur. "Marine Le Pen to borrow €6 million from father's lender." *Politico EU.* Dec. 31, 2016.

59 Tom McTague. "Marine Le Pen: Trump's election is a 'political revolution.'" *Politico EU.* Nov. 13, 2016.

60 Jasper Jackson. "Andrew Marr defends Remembrance Sunday Marine Le Pen interview." *The Guardian.* Nov. 13, 2016.

61 Nina Siegal. "Geert Wilders, Dutch Politician, Distracts From Hate-Speech Trial With More Vitriol." *The New York Times.* Oct. 31, 2016.

62 Nina Siegal. "Geert Wilders, Dutch Far-Right Leader, Is Convicted of Inciting Discrimination." *The New York Times.* Dec. 9, 2016.

63 Anna Holligan. "Dutch race hate row engulfs presenter Sylvana Simons." *BBC News, The Hague*. Nov. 25, 2016.

64 "'Disgusting' video circulates, showing Sylvana Simons as lynching victim." *Dutch News.Nl*. Nov. 21, 2016.

65 "Sylvana Simons should get out of politics, says Wilders." *Dutch News. Nl*. Nov. 23, 2016.

66 Janene Pieters. "Sylvana Simons Launched New Party Weeks Before Leaving DENK: Report." *NL Times*. Dec. 29, 2016.

67 Gregor Aisch, Adam Pearce, Bryant Rousseau. "How Far is Europe Swinging to the Right?" *The New York Times*. Dec. 5, 2016.

68 "Hungary migrant ban narrowly fails in parliamentary vote." *The Guardian*. Nov. 8, 2016.

69 David Crouch. "The rise of the anti-immigrant Sweden Democrats: 'We don't feel at home any more, and it's their fault.'" *The Guardian*. Dec. 13, 2014.

70 Supra note 67.

71 "Angela Merkel: Full-face veil must be banned in Germany." *Aljazeera*. Dec. 7, 2016.

72 "Paralympian tells of train toilet 'humiliation.'" *BBC News*, Jan. 3, 2017.

73 "'Wheelchair v buggy': Disabled man wins Supreme Court case." *BBC News*, Jan. 18, 2017.

74 "Wakefield wheelchair user refused space on bus." *BBC News*. Jan. 30, 2017.

75 Mark Brown. "Disabled people are to be 'warehoused.' We should be livid." *The Guardian*. Jan. 25, 2017.

76 Amelia Hill. "Winterbourne View care home staff jailed for abusing residents." *The Guardian*. Oct. 26, 2012.

77 "Reality Check: What has the EU meant for disability rights?" *BBC News*. Jun. 22, 2016.

78 European Commission."Disabilities: proposal for an Accessibility Act—frequently asked questions." Dec. 2, 2015.

79 "EU: A Commitment to Disability Rights." *Human Rights Watch*. Dec. 30, 2010.

80 "Convention on the Rights of Persons with Disabilities (CRPD). United Nations. https://www.un.org/development/desa/disabilities/convention-on-the-rights-of-persons-with-disabilities.html

CPSIA information can be obtained
at www.ICGtesting.com
Printed in the USA
LVHW081305241021
701372LV00011B/436

9 781941 960066